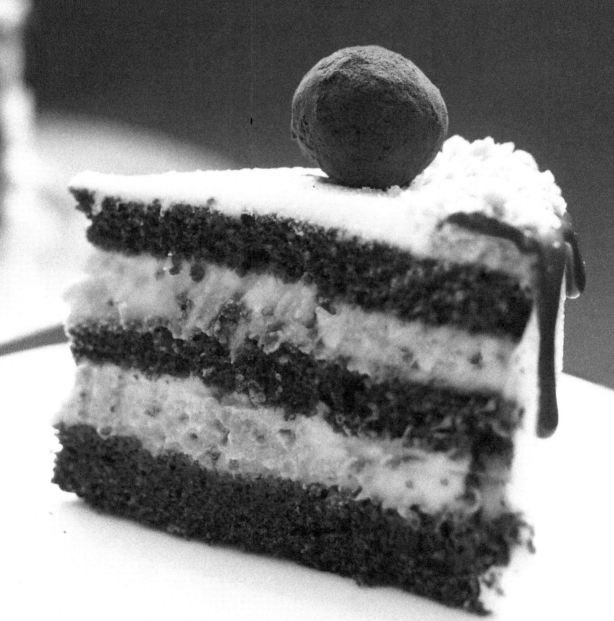

Delicious

VEGAN DESSERT

250 RECIPES FOR CAKES, COOKIES, PUDDINGS, CANDIES, AND MORE!

JOANNA J. WOOD

CHAPTER 8: NATURE'S CANDY: REFINED SUGAR–FREE TREATS…..293

Chapter 1

HOMEMADE BASICS

ALMOND MILK

There are lots of non dairy milks to choose from, but almond milk is easy to make. While there are many packaged options available, it's really easy to make yourself—and the bonus is there are no additives or any extra ingredients, plus the flavor is much richer than store-bought.

2 cups raw almonds
6 cups water

- Blend almonds and water in high-speed blender for about 7 minutes, or until well mixed into a thick liquid. Strain through a cheesecloth. Will keep in the fridge for 3 to 5 days.

You can discard the almond pulp or use it for a flour replacement or a protein fix in your morning smoothies. For flour replacement: Preheat oven to 375°F. Spread an even, thin layer of almond pulp onto an ungreased cookie sheet and bake for 10 to 12 minutes, or until lightly toasted. To dry using a dehydrator, spread the pulp onto a dehydrator sheet in a thin even layer and dehydrate at 130°F, for 5 hours, or until completely dry.

SIMPLE SYRUP

YIELD: 1¼ CUPS

It may just be sugar and water, but keeping a jar of simple syrup around will make for effortless cocktails, mocktails, coffee drinks, and more! This lasts indefinitely if stored in the fridge. If it begins to crystallize, simply warm again over the stove until once again dissolved.

1 cup sugar
½ cup water

- Over medium heat in a small saucepan, warm the ingredients just until the sugar has dissolved completely and the mixture turns from cloudy to mostly clear. Remove from heat before it reaches a boil. Let cool completely. Use as needed in recipes requiring simple syrup. Store in an airtight container in the refrigerator for up to 4 weeks.

DATE SYRUP

YIELD: 1½ CUPS

This makes a fantastic refined sugar–free sweetener that can be used in place of sugar or agave in many recipes. Keep a jar of this around to add to smoothies or plain non dairy yogurt in the mornings.

20 Medjool dates
Water to soak
1⅓ cups additional water

- Place the dates into a medium bowl. Cover with water and top with a salad plate. Let soak for 8 hours, drain, and replace the water, and then allow the dates to soak an additional 4 to 6 hours.

- Drain the dates completely and then remove the seeds and tops of the dates. Place into a blender along with 1⅓ cups water and blend until extremely smooth, scraping down the sides often.

- Store in an airtight container in the refrigerator for up to 1 month.

THE BESTEST NUT BUTTER
YIELD: 3 CUPS

Peanuts are the star of the show below, but this method works well with other roasted nuts, which comes in handy with a peanut allergy. Try toasted or raw almonds, cashews, or sunflower seeds instead. Even though nut butters are widely available in pretty much every grocery store in the United States, I think homemade is much tastier, and it's so much cheaper. And, it's easy! So easy, in fact, that you may wonder why you hadn't tried it sooner.

3 cups dry roasted peanuts, unsalted (or nuts or seeds of your choice)
1 teaspoon salt, or to taste
1 teaspoon vanilla extract

- Place the peanuts into a food processor and blend until very smooth, about 7 minutes, scraping down the sides of the bowl as needed. Add the salt and vanilla extract and mix well. Store in an airtight container for up to 3 months.

APPLE CIDER VINEGAR

YIELD: 2 GALLONS

Apple cider vinegar is one of those things that is just *so* much better homemade and can be made much cheaper at home than store-bought. All it takes is some apples and a lot of patience (like 2 months), but the end result is well worth the wait. And, don't be afraid of the gelatinous "mother" or the "yeasties" that float in the jar ... that's what makes the vinegar good! You'll need a 2-gallon glass jar or vessel with a wide mouth, as well as a piece of cheesecloth, about 16 × 16 inches, and a rubber band.

10 apples, chopped roughly into large chunks: seeds, stems, and all
¼ cup sugar
Water

- Place the apples into the large jar, pushing down gently with a ladle to pack the apples in. You can also use a clean saucer or small dish to weight down the apples inside the vessel. Next add in the sugar and then cover the apples with water so that they are completely submerged. Cover with the cheesecloth and then secure with a rubber band. This keeps the critters out but still allows air to help the process along. Place the jar carefully into a cool dark place for 1 week.

- Strain the apples from the vinegar and replace the cheesecloth. At this point you may transfer it to a different container, or several. Just be sure the containers are totally clean. Cap again with cheesecloth and rubber band and place back into a cool dark place for 6 to 8 more weeks. And that's it! You have the best darned vinegar money doesn't have to buy. You can bottle it and store as you would any bottle of vinegar. Store in an airtight container for 6 months to 1 year and beyond.

To sterilize containers, a good scrubbing with very hot soapy water, a hot rinse, and preferably a run through the dishwasher—complete with dry cycle—works perfectly.

VANILLA EXTRACT
YIELD: 5 CUPS

Although vanilla extract is fairly easy to come by, the stuff made at home is superior in flavor and will last virtually forever. I like to make up a big batch at once and bottle to give away to friends. Dark vanilla extract bottles work well for storing. Simply scrub off the labels and replace them with new!

5 cups bourbon (vodka works well, too)
12 vanilla beans, split

- Pour 5 cups of bourbon into a clean jar or bottle. Place the vanilla beans into the bottle of bourbon and reseal tightly. Place in cool dark place, such as a pantry, and store for 3 months. After three months, you can either use it straight from the bottle or bottle individually, leaving at least 1 vanilla bean in each bottle. As the bottle becomes empty, replace with more bourbon. After one year, replace the vanilla beans with new. Store in airtight container.

SWEET FACT

Vanilla beans are the second most expensive spice after saffron because growing and harvesting the beans is incredibly labor intensive.

SWEET CASHEW CREAM

YIELD: 5 CUPS

This recipe makes a fantastic substitute for dairy-based cream cheeses, whipped cream, and more. Store in an airtight container in the refrigerator for up to 2 weeks. Cashew cream can also be frozen and thawed for later use, with little effect on flavor or color. Just thaw in the fridge overnight before using.

4 cups raw cashews
1 cup water
1 teaspoon vanilla extract
3 tablespoons maple syrup or agave
⅛ teaspoon salt

- Before making, place the cashews into a large bowl and cover with 1 inch of water. Let soak 2 to 4 hours and then rinse well. Place cashews into a food processor along with the water, vanilla extract, maple syrup, and salt. Blend until smooth, scraping down sides as needed.

- Continue to blend, about 7 minutes, until very smooth and creamy. Use as a topping for a variety of treats as you would whipped cream, or as directed in recipes. Store in an airtight container in the refrigerator up to 1 week.

MASCARPONE

YIELD: 1 CUP

True mascarpone is a light, dairy-based cream cheese that has an ever-so- slightly sweet taste. In this version, I've used cashews in place of dairy. Feel free to use your own homemade margarine or coconut oil in this mascarpone. This spread can be stirred into your favorite puddings for an extra dose of creamy, or sandwich in between cake layers for a remarkable filling, such as the Tiramisu.

1 cup raw cashews
2 tablespoons non dairy margarine or coconut oil (add ¼ teaspoon salt if coconut oil is used)
1 tablespoon non dairy milk
1 tablespoon confectioners sugar

- Place the cashews in a bowl and cover with 3 cups of water; soak for 6 hours. Drain the cashews and rinse well. Place the soaked cashews into a food processor and blend until pasty, about 2 minutes, scraping down the sides often. Add the margarine, non dairy milk, and confectioners sugar and blend an additional 5 minutes, again, scraping the sides often, until a fluffy mixture is made. Store in an airtight container in the refrigerator for up to 5 days.

SWEETENED WHIPPED COCONUT CREAM

This whipped cream could not be easier. Stash a few cans of coconut milk in your fridge so you are ready to rock when the need arises for whipped cream. Also, use the best-quality coconut milk you can, and be sure it's full fat—with this recipe, quality counts.

1 (13.5-ounce) can full-fat (organic is best) coconut milk
1 tablespoon confectioners sugar, or 1 teaspoon powdered stevia

- Before you attempt to whip your coconut cream, place the can of coconut milk in your refrigerator and chill overnight. Flip the can upside down and open. Drain all liquid from the can (use it in smoothies or recipes that call for non dairy milk) until you are left with just the thick white cream from the can. Place the cream and confectioners sugar into a sturdy mixing bowl, and using a whisk attachment, whip until fluffy. Use immediately.

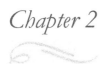

Chapter 2

KILLER CAKES AND TOPPINGS

Cakes are probably the most iconic celebration foods, being the ultimate centerpiece at birthdays and weddings, but I enjoy baking them "just because" every now and again, too. On the following pages, you'll find all you need to make the perfect cake, whether it be for a small wedding or a simple Sunday brunch.

CAKE BASICS

PREPPING AND ICING A LAYER CAKE

Making Layers Even

Ever bake a cake and once decorated, find it's a bit "rounder" than you anticipated? I'm here to let you know that it's not you—it's the nature of the cake! Unless cakes have been leveled, if you try and stack them, you'll end up with a fairly uneven mound of cake that slopes on the sides, which, although tasty, isn't the most aesthetically appealing. Baking bands come in handy, and I absolutely recommend them if you're trying to tackle large projects, such as multi layered cakes.

To make perfectly even layers, be sure to divide your batter evenly among pans. Use baking bands (soaked in water and then squeezed) to increase the odds of even baking. Once the cakes have baked, let them cool in the pans for about 30 minutes. After they are slightly cooled, gently slide a knife around the edges of the cake pan to release, and once the cakes have completely cooled, invert each one once onto a plate and then reposition it so that the top of the cake is facing up. Basically, you're flipping both cakes out of the pans and just making sure the bottom is on the bottom and top is on the top.

Use a long serrated knife to slice off just the tops of the cake so that both cake rounds appear very level. Use excess cake for crumbs … or just eat it! Now your cake is ready to be decorated!

CRUMB COAT

The scenario: You bake a fabulous cake and a perfectly complementary frosting, and you are so excited to show it off to your family and/or friends. But, once frosted, you are devastated to find that you have speckled your entire cake with pebbles of cake crumbs rather than a silky smooth layer of frosting. This is a common problem, friend, and it can be remedied. Crumb coat to the rescue!

For an Easy Crumb Coat

Use a small portion of your frosting to create a thin layer of frosting—cover each layer without worrying about keeping crumbs out of the icing; that's what this step is for! Crumb it up.

Now, place one of the layers onto a steady cake dish or icing plate.

Be sure to top each layer liberally with frosting and press gently to set the filling in between cakes. Repeat with as many layers as you have. Freeze the cake briefly, about 15 minutes, or until frosting has totally hardened.

Now you're ready for the final coat of frosting! Frost the entire cake again with a thick layer of frosting and garnish with any fancy piping that you can dream up.

LAYER AND SHEET CAKES

DEVIL'S FOOD CAKE

YIELD: ONE 9 × 13-INCH CAKE OR 12 CUPCAKES

A classic recipe for birthday parties and other celebrations, this version is as close to authentic, in taste and texture anyhow, as you can get. The surprise ingredient is tahini, the sesame seed paste commonly used in savory dishes like hummus.

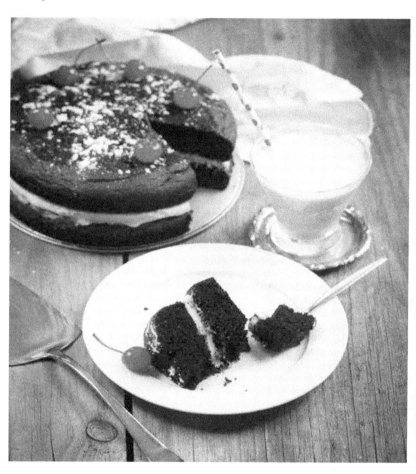

1¼ cups sorghum flour

¾ cup extra-dark cocoa powder

½ cup potato starch

¼ cup buckwheat flour

¼ cup sweet white rice flour

2 teaspoons xanthan gum

2 teaspoons baking soda

1 teaspoon baking powder

¼ teaspoon salt

½ cup olive oil

1½ cups sugar

2 tablespoons tahini

1 cup extra-strong coffee, cold

1 cup coconut milk

2 tablespoons apple cider vinegar

- Preheat oven to 350°F and grease and lightly flour a 9 × 13-inch cake pan or line 12 cupcake tins with paper liners.
- In medium bowl, combine sorghum flour, cocoa powder, potato starch, buckwheat flour, sweet white rice flour, xanthan gum, baking soda, baking powder, and salt. Whisk well to make sure everything is completely combined.
- In large mixing bowl, combine the olive oil, sugar, and tahini. Add one- third of the flour mix and stir until well combined. Mix in the coffee and coconut milk and the remaining flour mixture a little at a time until all has been incorporated. Stir in the vinegar until the batter is smooth and fluffy.
- Spread the cake batter into a prepared cake pan, or drop about ½ cup of batter into each cupcake liner. Bake for 27 to 30 minutes for sheet cake or cupcakes, or until knife inserted into the middle of the cake comes out clean. Let cool completely before frosting. Store covered for up to 3 days.

GERMAN CHOCOLATE CAKE

YIELD: 1 CAKE

The name "German Chocolate Cake" is actually a corruption of "German's Chocolate Cake" … meaning the "German's" chocolate bar that was named after their creator, Baker's Chocolate Company employee Sam German. Somewhere along the way, this dessert became known as German Chocolate Cake, even though it is quite American. Whatever you call it, it's tender and lighter in color than traditional chocolate cake; this recipe utilizes chocolate pieces rather than cocoa powder to give it that chocolaty flavor. You can also bake these as cupcakes, just reduce the baking time to 25 minutes, or until a knife inserted into the center comes out clean. Top with recommended icing.

¾ cup non dairy chocolate pieces or chips

¾ cup water, plus 4 tablespoons water

2 tablespoons flaxseed meal

1 ¼ cups brown rice flour

½ cup teff flour

2 teaspoons xanthan gum

1 cup potato starch

¼ cup tapioca flour

1 teaspoon baking powder

1 teaspoon baking soda

¾ teaspoon salt

1 cup non dairy margarine

1 ¾ cups sugar

1 teaspoon vanilla extract

½ cup non dairy milk

2 tablespoons apple cider vinegar

- Preheat oven to 350°F. Lightly grease and dust with cocoa powder two 9- inch round cake pans.

- In a small saucepan over medium-low heat, heat the chocolate and ¾ cup water until the chocolate is melted, stirring often. Remove from heat and set aside.

- In a small bowl, combine the flaxseed meal and 4 tablespoons water and let rest for 5 minutes, until gelled.

- In a large bowl, sift together the brown rice flour, teff flour, xanthan gum, potato starch, tapioca flour, baking powder, baking soda, and salt.

- Add the margarine, sugar, vanilla extract, and nondairy milk to the chocolate mixture and stir well to combine. Mix into the flour mixture along with the prepared flaxseed meal. Stir well, at least fifty strokes or 1 minute, and then stir in the vinegar.

- Divide the cake batter evenly between the two cake pans and bake for 25 to 30 minutes, or until knife inserted into the center comes out clean.

- Let cool completely, invert from pan, and then top each layer with German Chocolate Icing. Store covered for up to 3 days.

MARBLED CAKE

YIELD: 10 SERVINGS

This gorgeous cake needs no frosting in my opinion, as it offers plenty of sweet, sweet, goodness all by its lonesome. Plus, served undressed is the best way to show off its striking swirls.

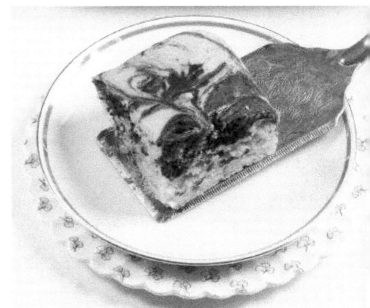

¾ cup white rice flour

½ cup brown rice flour

¾ cup besan/chickpea flour

1 cup potato starch

1½ teaspoons xanthan gum

2½ teaspoons baking powder

1 teaspoon baking soda

1 cup sugar

1 teaspoon salt

¾ cup olive oil

2 cups very cold water

2 tablespoons lemon juice

¼ cup cocoa powder

- Preheat oven to 350°F. Lightly grease an 8 × 8-inch cake pan. In a large bowl, whisk together the rice flours, besan, potato starch, xanthan gum, baking powder, baking soda, sugar, and salt. Add the olive oil, water, and lemon juice and stir well to achieve a very smooth batter.

- Pour about one-third of the batter into a bowl and whisk in the cocoa powder until evenly blended. Spread the yellow cake batter into the prepared baking pan and then drop dollops of the chocolate batter onto the yellow. Use a butter knife to gently swirl the two batters together into a loose and even pattern.

- Bake the cake for 35 to 40 minutes, or until a knife inserted into the middle comes out clean. Let cool before slicing with a serrated knife. Store covered for up to 3 days.

When marbling the batter, be sure to go the whole width of the cake to get the deepest variegation of contrast between the yellow and chocolate swirls. And don't overdo it! A little swirl goes a long way, and too much will muddy the pattern.

PINEAPPLE CHERRY UPSIDE-DOWN CAKE

YIELD: 8 SERVINGS

This cake is a favorite for many. ional birthday cake. It definitely increases the appeal that the cake makes its own icing!

⅔ cup cold non dairy margarine

¾ cup sugar

1 teaspoon vanilla extract

⅓ cup tapioca flour

½ teaspoon sea salt

1 teaspoon xanthan gum

3 teaspoons baking powder

¼ cup agave

2 cups besan/chickpea flour

1 cup pineapple juice

½ cup non dairy milk (unsweetened)

4 tablespoons softened margarine

½ cup brown sugar

7 pineapple rings, canned or fresh

7 maraschino cherries

- Preheat oven to 350°F and lightly grease the sides of an 8-inch springform pan.

- In a large mixing bowl, cream together the ⅔ cup margarine and sugar until fluffy. Mix in the vanilla extract, tapioca flour, sea salt, xanthan gum, baking powder, and agave until blended. Add the besan a little bit at a time, alternating with the pineapple juice, until all of each has been added. Whisk in the nondairy milk and mix until the cake batter is very smooth, at least fifty strokes. If you are using an electric mixer, let it run on medium for about 1 minute. (The batter will taste unpleasant due to the raw chickpea flour!)

- Spread the additional 4 tablespoons margarine onto the bottom of the springform pan, covering completely. Evenly sprinkle on the brown sugar and arrange the pineapple slices to fit snugly onto the bottom of the springform pan. Place the maraschino cherries into the holes of the pineapple rings for a pop of color. Spread the cake batter gently over the pineapples and place onto the middle oven rack with a large baking pan placed underneath to catch any drips.

- Bake for about 50 to 55 minutes, or until a knife inserted into the middle comes out clean. The edges will be very dark brown, but the middle should be bright and golden. Let the cake cool in the pan for 20 to 30 minutes before releasing the springform and inverting the cake onto a plate. Serve warm or room temperature. Store covered for up to 3 days.

OLIVE OIL CAKE

YIELD: 1 CAKE, ABOUT 8 SERVINGS

This moist and dense cake is a classic Italian American dessert and features the flowery undertones of olive oil rather than coconut oil or margarine. Serve after a delicious plate of pasta and hearty salad, along with a scoop of gelato.

1 cup superfine brown rice flour
½ cup potato starch
¼ cup tapioca flour
1 teaspoon xanthan gum
1 teaspoon salt
2 teaspoons baking powder
1 cup sugar
3 tablespoons lemon juice
¾ cup olive oil
½ cup + 2 tablespoons non dairy milk
Powdered sugar, for dusting

- Preheat oven to 350°F. Lightly grease and (brown rice) flour an 8-inch round cake pan.

- In a large bowl, whisk together the superfine brown rice flour, potato starch, tapioca flour, xanthan gum, salt, baking powder, and sugar. Add in the lemon juice, olive oil, and nondairy milk and whisk until very smooth. Spread the batter into the prepared cake pan and bake for 40 minutes, or until lightly golden brown on edges and a knife inserted into the center comes out clean. Let cool before dusting lightly with powdered sugar and cut using a serrated knife. Store covered for up to 3 days.

BANANA CAKE

YIELD: ONE 2-LAYER CAKE

If you love bananas, you'll adore this cake. I especially enjoy it paired with a Fluffy Chocolate Frosting or Dark Chocolate Ganache.

3 large very ripe bananas (peels should be brown)
⅔ cup olive oil
1 cup sugar
⅓ cup brown sugar
1 teaspoon vanilla extract
1 teaspoon salt
1½ cups brown rice flour
¾ cup potato starch
⅓ cup tapioca flour
1 teaspoon xanthan gum
2 teaspoons baking powder
2 teaspoons baking soda
½ cup plain non dairy yogurt
3 tablespoons apple cider vinegar

- Preheat oven to 350°F and lightly grease and (brown rice) flour two 8-inch round baking pans.

- In a large bowl, mix up the bananas until they are well mashed. Beat in the olive oil, sugars, and vanilla extract until smooth. Gradually add in the rest of the ingredients, mixing well after each addition. Spread batter between the two prepared baking pans and bake on the center rack for about 30 to 35 minutes, or until a knife inserted into the center comes out clean. Let cool in pans for about 15 minutes, then gently run a knife around the edges of the pans to release. Invert the cakes onto a wire cooling rack and allow to cool completely before frosting. Once cooled, follow the directions for Prepping and Icing a Layer Cake. Simply cover the tops of one cake with frosting, sandwich with another cake, and top the second layer with frosting. Store in airtight container or cake dish for up to 3 days.

This recipe also makes a delicious sheet cake. Simply grease and lightly flour a 9 × 13-inch pan, spread the prepared batter evenly, and bake for 30 to 35 minutes, or until a knife inserted into the middle comes out clean.

CUPCAKES

BOURBON CARAMEL CUPCAKES

YIELD: 12 CUPCAKES

Bourbon is one of my absolute favorite flavors because it pairs so perfectly with my other favorite flavors, vanilla and brown sugar. These bad boys tout all three flavors and make one heck of a fancy addition to a dessert tray. Not so keen on bourbon? You can replace it with apple cider or nondairy milk.

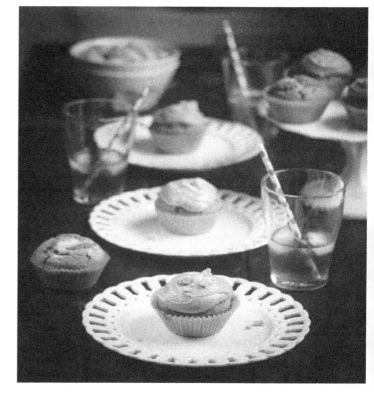

1¼ cups superfine brown rice flour

¾ cup sorghum flour

¾ cup potato starch

¼ cup sweet white rice flour

1½ teaspoons xanthan gum

2 teaspoons baking powder

1 teaspoon baking soda

1 teaspoon salt

¾ cup olive oil

1 cup brown sugar

⅓ cup sugar

2 tablespoons molasses

2 teaspoons vanilla extract

1 tablespoon ground chia seed mixed with ¼ cup water

½ cup bourbon

1 cup ice-cold water

- Preheat oven to 350°F. Line 12 muffin tins with paper liners.

- In a medium bowl, whisk together the brown rice flour, sorghum flour, potato starch, sweet white rice flour, xanthan gum, baking powder, baking soda, and salt.

- In a separate, larger bowl, combine the olive oil, sugars, molasses, 1 teaspoon of the vanilla extract, and chia mixture. Add a little bit of the flour mixture, the bourbon, and a little bit of the cold water plus the remaining teaspoon of vanilla extract and mix until smooth. Repeat with the flour mixture and the water until all of each has been incorporated completely. Mix the batter on high speed for 1 minute using an electric mixer, or about fifty strokes by hand.

- Drop ⅓ cup of batter into each prepared cupcake tin and bake for 25 to 30 minutes, or until a knife inserted into the middle comes out clean. Let cool completely before frosting with Caramel Frosting. Store covered for up to 2 days.

CLASSIC YELLOW CUPCAKES

YIELD: 24 CUPCAKES

Perfect for birthday parties, especially when paired with Fluffy Chocolate Frosting for a classic combo.

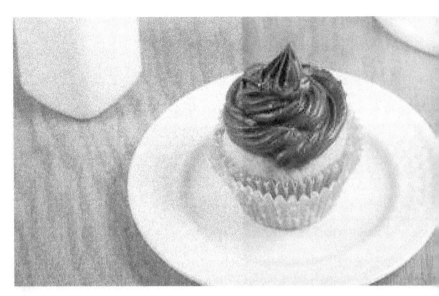

¾ cup white rice flour

½ cup brown rice flour

¾ cup besan/chickpea flour

¼ cup sweet white rice flour

¾ cup potato starch

1½ teaspoons xanthan gum

3 teaspoons baking powder

1 teaspoon baking soda

1 teaspoon vanilla

¾ cup melted non dairy margarine

1¼ cups sugar

1¼ cups canned coconut milk

1 cup water

2½ tablespoons apple cider vinegar

- Preheat oven to 350°F. Line 24 muffin tins with paper liners, or lightly grease and (brown rice) flour the individual cups.

- In a large bowl, whisk together the white rice flour, brown rice flour, besan, sweet white rice flour, potato starch, xanthan gum, baking powder, and baking soda. Gradually stir in the rest of the ingredients, as they are ordered, and whisk until very smooth. Drop a little less than ⅓ cup batter into the prepared baking trays and bake for about 27 minutes, or until knife inserted into the center comes out clean. Remove cupcakes from the pan and let them cool completely on a rack before frosting. Store covered in airtight container for up to 2 days.

This recipe can also be used to make a sheet cake; bake about 10 to 15 minutes longer, just until a knife inserted into the middle comes out clean.

BOSTON CREAM PIE CUPCAKES

YIELD: 12 CUPCAKES

This tender sponge cake with a tangy filling and topped with ganache is a tribute to the classic dessert Boston Cream Pie. In my opinion, the tangy cream filling is the best part—which comes from the unlikely addition of mayo!

CAKE

1⅓ cups superfine brown rice flour

¼ cup sweet white rice flour

¾ cup potato starch

⅔ cup besan/chickpea flour

2 teaspoons xanthan gum

3 teaspoons baking powder

1 teaspoon baking soda

1 teaspoon salt

1½ cups packed brown sugar

¾ cup olive oil

1 cup coconut milk

1¼ cups very cold water

2½ tablespoons lemon juice

FILLING

⅓ cup non dairy margarine

2 cups confectioners sugar

1 tablespoon non dairy milk

1 tablespoon lemon juice

1 tablespoon non dairy mayonnaise, such as Vegenaise

½ teaspoon xanthan gum

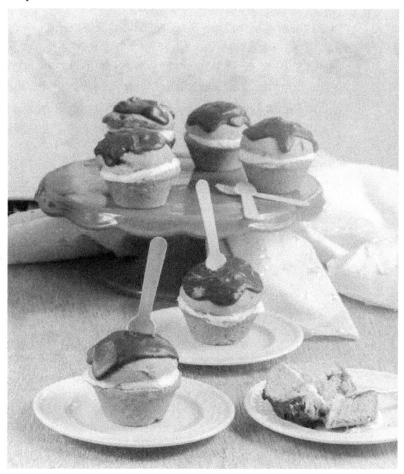

TOPPING

1 recipe <u>Dark Chocolate Ganache</u>

- Preheat oven to 350°F. Line a cupcake pan with 12 paper liners, or lightly grease and (brown rice) flour the individual cups.

- In a large mixing bowl, whisk together the brown rice flour, sweet white rice flour, potato starch, besan, xanthan gum, baking powder, baking soda, and salt.

- In the bowl of electric mixer, cream together the brown sugar, olive oil, and coconut milk. Gently add in the flour mixture, alternating with the water. Add the lemon juice and mix on high speed for about 1 to 2 minutes. Divide batter among the 12 muffin tins and bake for 35 minutes, or until puffed up high and golden brown, and knife inserted into center comes out clean. Let the cupcakes cool completely before filling and topping.

- To make the filling, combine all the ingredients using an electric mixer with a whisk attachment and whip until fluffy. Using a serrated knife, cut off tops of cupcakes just above the papers. Add about 2 tablespoons of filling and replace the top. Place cupcakes in the freezer on a flat surface a few minutes before topping with Dark Chocolate Ganache. Store loosely covered cupcakes in the refrigerator for up to 1 week.

CAPPUCCINO CUPCAKES

YIELD: 12 CUPCAKES

Let these cupcakes transport you to your favorite café with notes of deep dark espresso. The tender moist cake is a perfect complement to the recommended topping of the lighter-than-air Mocha Fluff frosting.

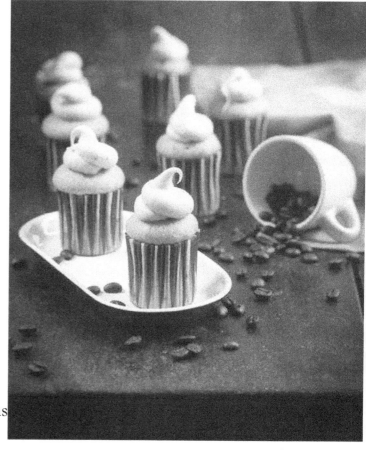

1 cup besan/chickpea flour
½ cup white rice flour
⅓ cup potato starch
¼ cup tapioca flour
1½ teaspoons baking powder
1 teaspoon salt
1 teaspoon xanthan gum
½ cup brown sugar
⅔ cup sugar
⅓ cup olive oil
3 teaspoons instant espresso powder
1½ cups water
1 tablespoon apple cider vinegar

- Preheat oven to 350°F and line 12 muffin tins with paper liners, or lightly spray with oil.

- In a large bowl, whisk together the besan, white rice flour, potato starch, tapioca flour, baking powder, salt, xanthan gum, and sugars. Make a well in the center of the flour mixture and add in the olive oil, espresso powder, water, and vinegar. Stir to mix well until batter is smooth. Fill cups about two-thirds full. Bake for 25 to 30 minutes, or until knife inserted into the center of one of the cupcakes comes out clean. Let the cupcakes cool completely on a rack before frosting. Store covered for up to 2 days.

- Top with Mocha-Fluff Frosting.

TUBE AND BUNDT CAKES

APPLE CAKE

YIELD: 1 CAKE

Apple Cake is perfect to bake when you want to "wow" without a lot of fuss. This cake is extra moist and flavorful with the addition of fresh apples. The secret is to slice the apples thinly and evenly. You don't want them too thin, but about ¼ × 1 × 1 inch is just right.

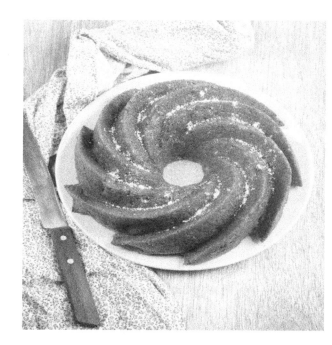

¾ cup brown rice flour

¾ cup besan/chickpea flour

½ cup potato starch

1 teaspoon xanthan gum

1 teaspoon baking powder

1 teaspoon baking soda

2 teaspoons cinnamon

¾ cup melted non dairy margarine

1 cup sugar

½ cup brown sugar

1 teaspoon vanilla extract

1 cup non dairy milk

1 tablespoon olive oil

4 apples, peeled, quartered, and sliced into thin pieces

- Preheat oven to 350°F. Lightly grease a standard-size nonstick tube pan.

- In a medium bowl, whisk together the brown rice flour, besan, potato starch, xanthan gum, baking powder, baking soda, and cinnamon.

- Make a well in the center and add the rest of the ingredients except the apples, stirring well after all has been added. Mix well, about fifty strokes. Fold in the apples until completely incorporated. Spread the cake batter into the prepared pan and bake for 65 to 70 minutes, or until a knife inserted into the center comes out clean. If using a different sized pan, check for doneness around the 40-minute mark by using the knife test.

- Let cool for 1 hour, and then run a knife around the outside and inside of the cake to loosen. Flip over onto a wire rack.

- Dust with confectioners sugar just before serving. Store covered up to 2 days.

This cake is so chock-full of apples that they become a big part of the cake's structure. Be sure to let your cake cool completely before cutting, or you may have an apple cake avalanche!

LEMON CAKE

YIELD: 1 BUNDT CAKE

Lemons always seem to put me in a good mood, and they dominate this cake. The tartness of the citrus in this cake pairs gorgeously with the airy texture. I recommend topping with Lemon Glaze or a simple dusting of confectioner's sugar.

1 cup non hydrogenated shortening

1½ cups sugar

⅓ cup + 1 tablespoon lemon juice

1 tablespoon lemon zest

1 cup besan/chickpea flour

⅓ cup brown rice flour

½ cup potato starch

½ cup tapioca flour

1 teaspoon xanthan gum

1 teaspoon salt

½ teaspoon baking powder

½ teaspoon baking soda

1 cup non dairy milk

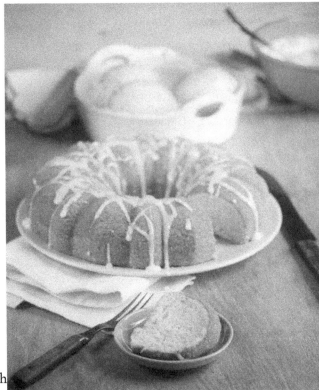

- Lightly grease a standard-size Bundt cake pan or two 8-inch round cake pans. Flour very lightly using white rice flour. Preheat oven to 350°F.

- In a large bowl of a stand mixer, combine the shortening, sugar, and lemon juice and mix until smooth and fluffy. Add in the lemon zest.

- In a separate bowl, whisk together the besan through the baking soda and then add the flour mixture into the sugar mixture along with the nondairy milk. Mix on low just until blended and then up the speed to high and mix for about 1 minute. The batter should be soft and fluffy.

- Spread the batter evenly into your prepared Bundt cake pan and bake on the center rack for 40 to 50 minutes, or until a knife inserted into the center comes out clean. Let cool for 1 hour and then run a knife around the outside and inside of the cake to loosen. Flip over onto a wire rack and let cool further. Top with Lemon Glaze. Store covered for up to 2 days.

CARROT APPLESAUCE CAKE

YIELD: 1 BUNDT CAKE

This cake is delightfully fragrant and tender with the comforting flavor of apples and a lovely subtle color from the carrots. Use any type of sugar you'd like. I love the standard evaporated cane juice … but light brown or coconut palm sugar would bake up nicely, too.

½ cup buckwheat flour
¾ cup sorghum flour
¾ cup potato starch
1 teaspoon xanthan gum
½ teaspoon sea salt
½ teaspoon baking powder
1½ teaspoons baking soda
1 teaspoon cinnamon
1¼ cups sugar
½ cup olive oil
1 cup applesauce (unsweetened)
2 tablespoons lemon juice
2 medium carrots, shredded

- Preheat oven to 350°F. Lightly grease and (sorghum) flour a standard-size tube or Bundt pan.

- In a large mixing bowl, whisk together the buckwheat flour, sorghum flour, potato starch, xanthan gum, sea salt, baking powder, baking soda, cinnamon, and sugar.

- Stir in the olive oil, applesauce, and lemon juice until well mixed and a thick batter has formed. Fold in the shredded carrots and evenly spread the batter into the prepared cake pan.

- Bake on the center rack for 40 to 45 minutes, or until a knife inserted into the center comes out clean. Let cool for 20 minutes before gently running a knife around the edge and inverting onto a flat serving dish. Store covered for up to 2 days.

HUMMINGBIRD BUNDT CAKE

YIELD: 1 BUNDT CAKE

A popular treat from the South, which is theorized to have originated in Jamaica, this cake was also widely known at one time as "The Cake That Doesn't Last." A fun play on the traditional Southern classic, this dessert takes the cake with all its scrumptious add-ins like pineapple, banana, and walnuts.

1¼ cups brown rice flour

¾ cup besan/chickpea flour

1 cup potato starch

1 teaspoon xanthan gum

2½ teaspoons baking powder

1 teaspoon baking soda

½ teaspoon salt

½ cup melted non dairy margarine

1 teaspoon cinnamon

1 cup sugar

3 very ripe bananas, mashed

1 cup pineapple juice

½ cup water

1 teaspoon vanilla extract

1⅓ cups small pineapple chunks

1 cup crushed pecans

Cream Cheese Frosting, glaze variation

- Lightly grease a standard-size Bundt pan.

- In a large bowl, whisk together the brown rice flour, besan, potato starch, xanthan gum, baking powder, baking soda, and salt. Stir in the margarine, cinnamon, sugar, bananas, pineapple juice, water, and vanilla extract and mix well using a whisk until smooth. Fold in the pineapple chunks. Sprinkle the pecans into the Bundt cake pan and pour the batter over the pecans. Bake for 70 minutes, or until a knife inserted into the cake comes out clean. Let cool in the pan for 20 minutes and invert onto a rack to cool completely. Store covered in the refrigerator for up to 3 days.

- Top with Cream Cheese Frosting, glaze variation.

RUM CAKE

This is a gem of a cake that my mother made often when I was a child, and that I didn't appreciate until I was a full-fledged adult. Although my mom's original recipe isn't gluten-free or vegan, I can assure you that this version is just as incredible.

CAKE
¾ cup white rice flour

½ cup brown rice flour

¾ cup besan/chickpea flour

1 cup potato starch

1½ teaspoons xanthan gum

2½ teaspoons baking powder

1 teaspoon baking soda

1 cup sugar

1 teaspoon salt

½ cup rum

1½ cups water

½ cup olive oil

3 tablespoons lime juice

1 cup chopped pecans or walnuts

RUM SAUCE
½ cup non dairy margarine

½ cup rum

½ cup water

1 cup sugar

- Preheat oven to 325°F and lightly grease a standard-size Bundt cake pan. In a large bowl, whisk together the flours, potato starch, xanthan gum, baking powder, baking soda, sugar, and salt.

- Make a well in the center of the flour mixture and add the rum, water, olive oil, and lime juice. Stir well until batter is very smooth. Sprinkle the chopped nuts onto the bottom of the Bundt cake pan and then spoon the batter on top of the nuts. Bake for 60 to 65 minutes on the middle rack of the oven, until risen and golden brown. Once the cake has finished baking, keep it in the pan while you make the rum sauce.

- For the sauce, in a small saucepan, combine the margarine, rum, water, and sugar. Bring

43

the mixture to a boil over medium heat, stirring often. Boil for 5 minutes and then gingerly drizzle the sauce onto the top of the cake while it is still sitting snugly in the pan. Let the cake rest for 45 minutes to 1 hour and then very carefully invert the cake onto a flat plate. Serve at room temperature. Store covered for up to 2 days.

Be sure to let this cake cool completely before handling, as it is very fragile while still warm.

LOAF CAKES AND BREADS

CLASSIC BANANA BREAD

YIELD: 1 LOAF

This is a version of that cake, minus the gluten and eggs. This banana bread pairs awfully well with a cup of crushed walnuts or pecans, so toss a few in the batter right before it hits the pan if you like your loaves a little nutty.

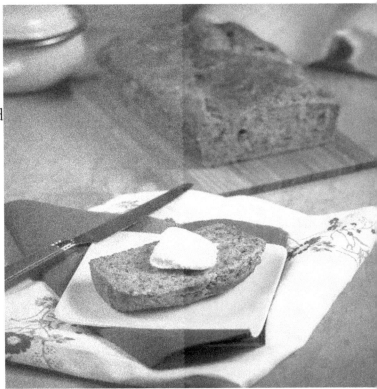

½ tablespoon ground chia seed

2 tablespoons water

¾ cup sugar

2 teaspoons bourbon or vanilla extract

4 very ripe medium bananas (skins should be mostly brown)

1 cup superfine brown rice flour

½ cup sorghum flour

½ cup cornstarch

¼ cup tapioca flour

1 teaspoon xanthan gum

1 teaspoon salt

1 teaspoon baking powder

1 teaspoon baking soda

- Preheat oven to 350°F and lightly grease a standard-size loaf pan with margarine or refined coconut oil.

- In a small bowl, mix together the chia seed with the water and let rest for 5 minutes until gelled.

- In a large bowl, use a potato masher to blend together the prepared chia "egg," sugar, bourbon, and bananas until smooth. Large lumps of banana aren't so good; small lumps are encouraged.

- In a separate smaller bowl, whisk together the remaining dry ingredients until blended. Gradually stir into the banana mixture until it comes together into a thick batter.

- Gently spoon the batter evenly into the prepared loaf pan and bake on the middle rack for 60 minutes, or until a knife inserted into the center comes out clean. Once baked, allow to cool for 10 minutes and then run a knife along the edges of the pan to loosen. Transfer to a wire rack to cool completely. Store covered in airtight container for up to 2 days.

VANILLA BEAN POUND CAKE

YIELD: 1 LOAF

Delightfully moist and simple, this cake is fantastic on its own and makes a lovely base for mix-ins, such as ½ cup of sliced almonds, dried berries, or chocolate chips.

1 cup sorghum flour

1 cup besan/chickpea flour

¼ cup tapioca flour

½ cup potato starch

2 teaspoons xanthan gum

2½ teaspoons baking powder

½ teaspoon salt

2 tablespoons melted coconut oil

1 tablespoon non dairy milk

¼ cup orange juice

2 cups granulated sugar

1 teaspoon vanilla extract

2 teaspoons ground chia seed mixed with 2 tablespoons water

2 tablespoons apple cider vinegar

1 teaspoon scraped vanilla bean (scraped from inside the pod)

- Preheat oven to 350°F and grease and lightly flour a standard-size metal loaf pan.

- In a large mixing bowl, whisk together the flours, potato starch, xanthan gum, baking powder, and salt until well blended. Add the rest of the ingredients and mix well until a thin, uniform batter forms. Pour it into the prepared loaf pan and bake for 50 minutes, undisturbed. Once finished cooking, turn the oven off, gently open the oven door a crack, and allow the cake to rest in the oven for an additional 45 minutes. Remove from the oven and cool completely before cutting with a serrated knife. Store covered for up to 2 days.

CHOCOLATE CHIP PUMPKIN BREAD

YIELD: 1 LOAF

A fun twist on an old favorite, chocolate chips add an extra touch of sweetness to this moist pumpkin bread. For an extra indulgent treat, use this as the bread base for the Bread Pudding recipe.

2 tablespoons flaxseed meal
4 tablespoons water
½ cup non dairy margarine
1½ cups sugar
1 cup canned pumpkin puree
¾ cup sorghum flour
⅓ cup buckwheat flour
⅓ cup potato starch
¼ cup sweet white rice flour
1 teaspoon xanthan gum
½ tablespoon baking powder
¾ teaspoon baking soda
⅛ teaspoon salt
1 cup non dairy chocolate chips

- Preheat oven to 350°F. In a small bowl, combine the flaxseed meal and water and let rest for 5 minutes, until gelled. Lightly grease and (sorghum) flour a standard-size glass loaf pan.

- In large mixing bowl, cream the margarine with the sugar and then incorporate the pumpkin. Stir in the prepared flaxseed meal.

- In a separate smaller bowl, whisk together the sorghum flour, buckwheat flour, potato starch, sweet rice flour, xanthan gum, baking powder, baking soda, and salt.

- Gradually incorporate the flour mixture into the pumpkin mixture and then mix well until a thick batter forms. Fold in the chocolate chips and spread into the prepared loaf pan.

- Bake in preheated oven for 70 to 75 minutes, or until a knife inserted into the center comes out clean. Store covered in airtight container for up to 2 days.

CINNAMON RAISIN BREAD

YIELD: 1 LOAF

This fragrant bread is a lovely addition to a tea party, with sweet cinnamon and plump raisins dotted throughout. This bread is exceptionally good toasted and slathered with Raspberry Chia Jam.

1 tablespoon active dry yeast

¼ cup sugar

1½ cups warm water, about 105°F

3 tablespoons coconut oil

1¼ cups buckwheat flour

¾ cup sorghum flour

2 teaspoons cinnamon

1 cup potato starch

½ cup tapioca flour

2 teaspoons xanthan gum

1 teaspoon salt

1½ cups raisins

¼ cup turbinado sugar

• Preheat oven to 450°F. Grease a standard-size loaf pan with olive oil.

• In a large bowl, combine the yeast with the sugar and water; proof until foamy, for about 5 minutes. Add the coconut oil.

• In a separate bowl, whisk together the buckwheat flour, sorghum flour, cinnamon, potato starch, tapioca flour, xanthan gum, and salt. Mix the dry ingredients in with the wet ingredients and stir just until blended. Fold in the raisins.

• Pat the dough evenly into the greased loaf pan. Lightly cover with a kitchen towel and allow to rest in a warm place for 1 hour. Sprinkle the top of the bread with the turbinado sugar. Bake the bread for 15 minutes, then reduce heat to 375°F and bake for an additional 30 to 35 minutes, or until the loaf sounds hollow when tapped.

• Let cool for 15 minutes and then remove from pan. Let cool completely before slicing with a serrated knife. Store covered in airtight container for up to 2 days.

OTHER CAKE TREATS

PUMPKIN ROLL

YIELD: 8 SERVINGS

This pumpkin roll freezes exceptionally well, allowing you to just take off a bit when a craving strikes and reserve an emergency stash for later. It's my go-to treat for a late night, early autumn sweet fix.

3 tablespoons flaxseed meal
6 tablespoons water
⅓ cup sorghum flour
2 tablespoons brown rice flour
1 tablespoon potato starch
¼ cup tapioca flour
1 teaspoon xanthan gum
1 teaspoon salt
1 teaspoon baking soda
1 cup sugar
½ teaspoon cinnamon
¼ teaspoon cloves
¼ teaspoon nutmeg
1 cup canned pumpkin puree
1 teaspoon lemon juice
1 recipe Cream Cheese Frosting

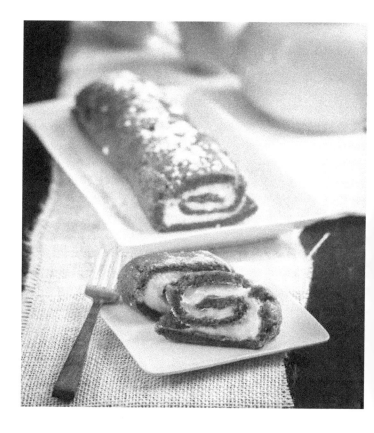

- Preheat oven to 375°F. Line a jelly roll pan with a large silicone baking mat or two sheets of parchment paper. Spray lightly with nonstick oil spray, such as PAM.

- Prepare your flaxseed "egg" mixture by mixing the flaxseed meal with the water and allowing it to rest for at least 5 minutes, or until thick.

- In a large bowl, whisk together all the dry ingredients and then add the pumpkin puree, lemon juice, and prepared flaxseed meal. Stir just until smooth and evenly mixed. Spread the mixture evenly into a rectangular shape on your prepared cookie sheet, about ½ inch thick. Bake for 14 minutes in preheated oven. Let cool for about 5 minutes, and then carefully flip out onto a large piece of plastic wrap on a flat surface. Sprinkle lightly to coat with confectioners sugar and then place a clean tea towel on top of the cake (or, coat one side of the towel with confectioners sugar and place sugar side down onto the cake). Roll up lengthwise, tea towel and all, and allow to cool about 20 minutes in a cool place (an open window during fall is perfect for this). Don't let it stay in the towel too long, or it may stick.

- Unroll the slightly cooled roll, and carefully remove the towel. Spread the icing in the middle of the cake and immediately reroll back up lengthwise. Dust with confectioners sugar. Refrigerate for at least 2 to 3 hours before serving. Store covered in airtight container in refrigerator for up to 1 week, or freeze for up to 3 months.

This recipe is best made on a dry day. Humid or rainy weather can cause the dough to become sticky.

STRAWBERRY SHORTCAKE

YIELD: 8 SHORTCAKES

Nothing says summertime like the taste of sweetened strawberries atop a delicate shortcake. Don't forget the whipped coconut cream! Feel free to adjust the amount of sugar depending on the natural sweetness of your berries. Use more or less sugar as needed.

SHORTCAKES

1½ cups superfine brown rice flour

¼ cup cornstarch

¼ cup tapioca flour

1 teaspoon xanthan gum

2½ teaspoons baking powder

⅓ cup sugar

½ cup cold non dairy margarine, cut into small pieces

½ cup non dairy milk

1 tablespoon flaxseed meal

2 tablespoons water

STRAWBERRY MIX

3 cups strawberries

½ cup sugar

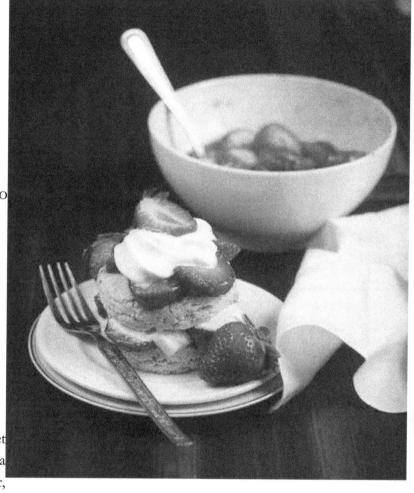

- Preheat oven to 400°F. Line a large baking sheet with parchment paper or a silicone mat. In a large bowl, whisk together the brown rice flour, cornstarch, tapioca flour, xanthan gum, baking powder, and sugar. Use your fingers to crumble in the margarine until the mixture is pebbly. Add the non dairy milk. Mix the flaxseed meal with the water and then stir into the mixture. Knead lightly to form a very soft dough. Roll dough between two sheets of parchment until half an inch thick and using a biscuit cutter, cut into 2-inch rounds. Place 2 inches apart and bake for 17 to 20 minutes, or until lightly golden brown on edges.

- Rinse and slice the strawberries and discard the greens or reserve for another use, such as smoothies or salad greens. Place the strawberries into a bowl and toss with sugar. Cover and let rest for 1 hour. Serve with shortcakes and Sweetened Whipped Coconut Cream with proportions of each to suit your fancy.

- Store cakes separately in airtight container for up to 2 days.

PETITS FOURS

YIELD: 24 CAKES

These take a little finesse and time to put together, but the end result is so fun, you'll want to do it all over again! These are an especially good choice to bring along to potlucks, or to serve at a dinner party, a la mode with a little Matcha Cashew Ice Cream, perhaps?

CAKE

2 cups sugar

1½ cups olive oil

3 teaspoons vanilla extract

1 teaspoon salt

2 teaspoons baking powder

1¾ cups sorghum flour

¼ cup besan/chickpea flour

½ cup tapioca flour

½ cup potato starch

2 teaspoons xanthan gum

1 cup non dairy milk

2 tablespoons vinegar

3 tablespoons lemon juice

FILLING

½ cup raspberry preserves

8 ounces Marzipan

GLAZE

1 recipe Lemon Glaze or Vanilla Glaze

2 ounces non dairy chocolate, melted, for drizzling

- Preheat oven to 350°F. Grease and (sorghum) flour a 9 × 13-inch baking pan.

- In a large mixing bowl, combine the sugar, olive oil, vanilla extract, and salt and mix until smooth. In a separate bowl, whisk together the baking powder, sorghum flour, besan, tapioca flour, potato starch, and xanthan gum. Add about 1 cup of the flour mixture to the sugar mixture and mix well, and then stir in the nondairy milk. Blend in the remainder of the flour mix and mix well, for about 1 minute or fifty-five strokes. Stir in the vinegar and lemon juice. Spread evenly into prepared baking pan.

- Bake at 350°F for 40 to 45 minutes, undisturbed, until knife inserted in middle comes out clean. Let cool for about 30 minutes and gently run a knife around the edge to release. Flip over onto a wire rack and let cool completely, for at least 2 hours.

- Once cake is cool, cut into 1 × 1-inch squares. Cut the squares in half, and then spread a bit of preserves (about ½ teaspoon) onto one of the cakes, and top with another cake to form a sandwich. Repeat until all cakes have been cut and sandwiched together.

- Place the marzipan in between two sheets of parchment paper and roll as thinly as possible without tearing the marzipan. Cut evenly into 1 × 1-inch squares and place one small square on top of the sandwiched cakes until all have been covered.

- Prepare the glaze and immediately dip the cakes into the glaze, one by one, and then place them onto a wire rack with a large cookie sheet underneath. Let the cakes harden briefly and then repeat with another layer. Drizzle with melted chocolate and let rest for at least 1½ hours, or until firm. Store covered in airtight container for up to 2 days.

CHERRY BOMBS

YIELD: 6 CAKES

I adore these little desserts. Crispy, fluffy, chewy cake is topped with caramelized cherries that deliver an explosion of flavor.

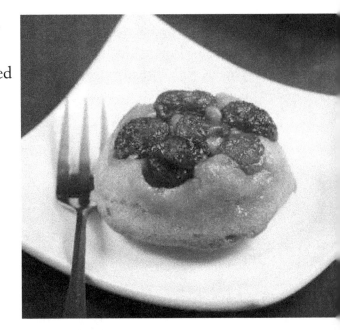

1½ teaspoons non dairy margarine or coconut oil

6 tablespoons turbinado sugar

2 cups whole sweet cherries, pitted, stems removed

½ cup besan/chickpea flour

¼ cup superfine brown rice flour

¼ cup potato starch

1 teaspoon baking powder

½ teaspoon xanthan gum

½ cup sugar

½ teaspoon salt

⅔ cup non dairy milk

¼ cup olive oil

2 tablespoons lime juice

- Preheat oven to 350°F and liberally grease a 6-count large muffin tin with the margarine, leaving about ¼ teaspoon spread evenly onto the bottom of the cups. Sprinkle the turbinado sugar into the muffin tin, 1 tablespoon evenly into each cup. Arrange the cherries to fit snugly into the bottoms of the tins, about six cherries per cup, pitted sides facing up.

- In a medium bowl, whisk together the besan, brown rice flour, potato starch, baking powder, xanthan gum, sugar, and salt. Stir in the nondairy milk, olive oil, and lime juice and beat until fluffy, about fifty strokes or 1 minute.

- Divide the batter evenly among the 6 cups and bake for 40 to 45 minutes, until golden brown on tops and baked through. Let cool for 5 minutes, and then gently scoop the cakes out with a large spoon, inverting onto a serving dish. Store covered in refrigerator for up to 2 days.

When choosing cherries, seek out plump and brightly colored fruits. Avoid any fruit that is bruised or damaged, as the bruised fruit tends to make the good fruit go bad quickly.

CHOCOLATE WHOOPIE PIES

YIELD: 12 PIES

A treat whose roots are from Maine, whoopie pies have grown increasingly popular over the years. They live somewhere in between a cake and a cookie and are traditionally stuffed with a fluffy frosting, but fill them with whatever you please, such as ganache or even a decadent jam.

PIES

1¼ cups brown rice flour

½ cup potato starch

¼ cup tapioca flour

⅓ cup cocoa powder

1 teaspoon xanthan gum

1 teaspoon baking soda

1 cup sugar

2 tablespoons flaxseed meal

4 tablespoons water

½ cup non dairy margarine, melted

¾ cup non dairy milk

FILLING

1 recipe Fluffy Bakery-Style Frosting

- Preheat oven to 350°F. Line a cookie sheet with a silicone baking mat or lightly grease.

- In a large bowl, whisk together all of the ingredients up until the flaxseed meal.

- In a small bowl, mix the flaxseed meal with the water and let rest for 5 minutes to form a gel.

- Mix in the prepared flaxseed, melted margarine, and nondairy milk and mix well to form a foamy batter.

- Drop by evenly rounded tablespoons onto the cookie sheet about 2 inches apart. Bake for 11 minutes and let cool completely before carefully removing from the cookie sheet. Once cookies are cooled, spread 2 tablespoons Fluffy Bakery-Style Frosting onto one of the cookies and then gently press another cookie on top and gently smoosh to combine. Repeat until all cakes have been assembled. Store covered in airtight container for up to 3 days.

A tasty berry-ation: Add a couple tablespoons Strawberry Preserves into the fluffy frosting to make Strawberry Chocolate Whoopie Pies.

TOPPINGS: FROSTINGS, GLAZES, AND SAUCES

MARSHMALLOW FONDANT

YIELD: COVERS ONE 2-LAYER CAKE

Fondant is one of those wonderful things that can help transform a cake from "meh" to "marvelous!" It is easy to use and can be made into multiple colors. You can also use fondant to make cute cut out shapes to paste onto your cake. Once you've covered your cake, roll out a thin layer and then cut out using cookie cutter—see Rolling Fondant. Lightly brush one side with water and paste it to the cake.

1 bag (10 ounces) vegan marshmallows, such as Dandies

¼ cup warm water

1 teaspoon vanilla extract (optional)

½ tablespoon refined coconut oil, plus ¼ cup for kneading and greasing

2 to 3 drops food coloring (optional)

1½ cups confectioner's sugar + about ½ cup extra for kneading

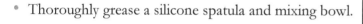

- Thoroughly grease a silicone spatula and mixing bowl.

- Place the marshmallows into a medium saucepan and heat over medium- low heat until sticky, for about 5 minutes, stirring often. Add the water, vanilla extract, ½ tablespoon coconut oil, and food coloring, if desired. Continue to cook over medium-low heat until completely smooth, for about 7 minutes, stirring often with the greased silicone spatula.

- Transfer to a very well greased mixing bowl. Carefully beat in 1½ cups confectioner's sugar until tacky. There most likely will be confectioner's sugar remaining in the bottom of the bowl. It's okay, just leave it.

- Using greased hands, remove from the bowl and knead in about ½ tablespoon coconut oil and more confectioner's sugar until the dough is no longer sticky. It should take quite a few small additions of confectioner's sugar, about ½ cup total, to get it to the right consistency.

- Wrap in plastic wrap and chill overnight. Remove the fondant from the refrigerator about 10 to 15 minutes before using. Store in airtight container in refrigerator for up to 2 weeks.

Rolling Fondant

Whether you use my recipe for Marshmallow Fondant, or opt for store-bought, such as Satin Ice brand, working with fondant is easier than it looks; in fact, I think it's the easiest way to make a spectacular-looking cake with little fuss. You simply need to have a few inexpensive tools on hand to make it look flawless.

Always keep a small container of coconut oil handy for greasing your hands as fondant tends to dry out quickly but can easily be saved by massaging a touch of coconut oil or shortening into it.

When working with fondant, I recommend having a few special tools on hand to make the experience easier. A fondant roller and rubber rolling rings are handy, as well as a fondant spatula, which will enable a smooth application onto your cake.

The most important tip I can offer is to make sure that the cake you are covering is even. Use a serrated knife to carve the cakes into even layers (usually only the very top needs to be trimmed) and fill in gaps with a little extra frosting. Use the method on to create a crumb coat, and, if desired, add a final layer of frosting to the outside of the cake. Now you are ready to cover the cake.

When rolling out fondant, be sure to roll out onto a very clean, flat, and lightly confectioner's sugared surface. Use plastic rings on a fondant roller to determine the thickness of your fondant, which will ensure an even layer on your cake. Use the fondant roller to help lift the rolled fondant and transfer it evenly onto the cake. Mend any tears or cracks with a touch of water and/or coconut oil. Finally, smooth out the cake with the fondant spatula, gently moving the spatula over the fondant in a circular motion to remove any large bumps or bubbles. You can insert a clean pin into any small bubbles to "pop" them before smoothing over, if needed. Seal edges with fondant balls or piped icing.

BUTTERCREAM FROSTING

YIELD: 4 CUPS

A standard in any dessert lover's arsenal, this recipe works exceptionally well with either margarine or coconut oil. If you opt for the latter, add a pinch of salt and keep slightly chilled.

6 tablespoons non dairy margarine or coconut oil (cold)
6 cups confectioners sugar
2 to 3 teaspoons vanilla extract
6 tablespoons non dairy milk
2 additional tablespoons softened non dairy margarine or coconut oil

- Cream together the 6 tablespoons margarine and about ½ cup of the confectioner's sugar. Gradually add in other ingredients, except the softened margarine. Once all the other ingredients have been combined and are fairly smooth, add in softened margarine.

- Mix on very high speed, using a whisk attachment, whipping until fluffy.

- Use immediately on cake, or chill in fridge for later use. If refrigerated, make sure you let it soften slightly by setting the icing out at room temperature just until it is softened enough to spread easily onto cake. If you find the icing too thick, add a touch more nondairy milk to thin. Store in airtight container in refrigerator for up to 2 weeks.

FLUFFY BAKERY-STYLE FROSTING

YIELD: 2 CUPS

Use this classic frosting to fill Whoopie Pies, cupcakes, and more. This frosting can easily be made up to 1 week ahead of time and stored in the refrigerator before using. Be sure to thaw to room temperature before using.

2 cups confectioners sugar
1 cup non hydrogenated shortening
¼ cup non dairy margarine

- Beat together the ingredients in an electric mixing bowl, or by hand, until fluffy. Store refrigerated and allow to warm slightly at room temperature before piping or spreading onto cakes or cookies. Store in airtight container in refrigerator for up to 1 week.

CREAM CHEESE FROSTING

YIELD: 1¼ CUPS

A foolproof recipe with a tangy twist. Feel free to sub in 1 cup Sweet Cashew Cream + 1 teaspoon lemon juice in place of the vegan cream cheese. To make a drizzly glaze rather than a fluffy frosting, simply thin with 2 to 3 tablespoons nondairy milk and 1 teaspoon agave or corn syrup.

8 ounces nondairy cream cheese
2 cups confectioners sugar

- Make the icing by mixing the ingredients vigorously by hand, or using an electric mixer, until fluffy. Chill before using. Store in airtight container in refrigerator for up to 1 week.

FLUFFY CHOCOLATE FROSTING

YIELD: 2 CUPS

Better than the stuff from a can, but just as addictive. Top your favorite cupcakes or use as a filling in between cookies, like the Vanilla Wafers.

⅔ cup cocoa powder
⅓ cup non hydrogenated shortening
¼ cup softened non dairy margarine
¼ cup non dairy milk
2½ cups confectioner's sugar

- In a large mixing bowl fitted with a whisk attachment, combine the cocoa powder, shortening, and margarine until smooth. Gradually add the non dairy milk and confectioners sugar and then beat on high speed until fluffy, scraping down the sides as needed. Makes enough for one sheet cake; double recipe if making for a layer cake. Store in airtight container in refrigerator for up to 2 weeks.

GERMAN CHOCOLATE ICING
YIELD: TOPS 1 GERMAN CHOCOLATE CAKE

This sweet coconutty icing makes an apropos topper for German Chocolate Cake, but it's just as scrumptious in other applications as well! Try it atop a big scoop of Vanilla Soft Serve.

½ cup agave
¾ cup powdered sugar
2 tablespoons non dairy milk
1 cup pecans, finely chopped
2 tablespoons coconut oil, softened
2 cups sweetened shredded coconut

- In a medium bowl, whisk together the agave, powdered sugar, and nondairy milk until smooth. Add the rest of the ingredients and mix well. Spread onto cakes while they are still warm, or pipe onto cupcakes using a bag with no tip. Store in airtight container in refrigerator for up to 2 weeks.

CARAMEL FROSTING

YIELD: COVERS 12 CUPCAKES

This rich and velvety frosting is reminiscent of sweet and salty caramel candies, without the need to slave over the stove. Even though this frosting goes stunningly with the recommended Bourbon Caramel Cupcakes, this also tastes fantastic on chocolate cake. For an over-the-top treat, try it slathered on top of my Ultimate Fudgy Brownies, and sprinkled with toasted pecans.

2 cups confectioners sugar
½ teaspoon vanilla extract
1 tablespoon molasses
¼ cup non dairy milk
⅛ teaspoon salt
1 tablespoon non dairy margarine

- Combine all ingredients, in the order given, into a small electric mixing bowl and mix on high speed until smooth and tacky. Spread generously onto the tops of cooled cupcakes or layer cake. Store in airtight container in refrigerator for up to 2 weeks.

MOCHA-FLUFF FROSTING

YIELD: 1½ CUPS

This frosting is best used right after preparing, since as it cools, it hardens into a fantastically light and airy, candy-like topping.

1 cup vegan marshmallows, such as Dandies
1 tablespoon non dairy margarine
2 teaspoons instant espresso powder
2 cups confectioners sugar
1 tablespoon non dairy milk

- In a small saucepan, heat the marshmallows, margarine, and espresso powder over medium-low heat until the marshmallows and margarine have melted. Stir constantly and then immediately transfer into a mixing bowl equipped with a whisk attachment. Blend on low as you add in the sugar and nondairy milk and then increase speed to high and whip just until fluffy. Quickly transfer into a piping bag fitted with a large round tip and pipe onto cupcakes.

You can double the batch of this recipe and make a confection a lot like a vegan meringue. Just pipe onto parchment or waxed paper and let air-dry for about 6 hours.

VANILLA GLAZE

YIELD: 1 CUP

Particularly nice for glazing one-half of a Black and White Cookie, this glaze also works well for cakes, Blondies, and pretty much any treat you can think of.

1 cup confectioners sugar
1 tablespoon + 1 to 2 teaspoons non dairy milk
1½ teaspoons light corn syrup
⅛ teaspoon vanilla extract Dash salt

- In a small bowl, whisk all the ingredients together until very smooth, ensuring no lumps remain. Use immediately after making and let set for at least 1 hour before handling.

CHOCOLATE GLAZE

YIELD: 1 CUP

This super-easy glaze tastes just like the icing on popular chocolate snack cakes and makes a perfect alternate glaze for Petits Fours.

⅓ cup melted non dairy chocolate coins or chips
1 teaspoon coconut oil
⅓ cup confectioners sugar
1 teaspoon corn syrup
1 tablespoon non dairy milk

- In a small bowl, whisk together the chocolate and coconut oil until smooth. Gradually add the confectioner's sugar, corn syrup, and nondairy milk, stirring continuously to blend. Stir vigorously until very smooth. Use immediately to top cookies and cakes. Let set for 2 hours before handling.

LEMON GLAZE

YIELD: 1 CUP

Perfect atop Lemon Cake or drizzled onto Sugar Cookies, this glaze sets quickly and should be prepared right before using.

1 large lemon, sliced thinly
1 cup sugar
1½ to 2 cups confectioners sugar
1 teaspoon corn syrup

- In a 2-quart saucepan over medium heat, bring the lemon slices and sugar to a gentle boil and let cook for 1 minute. Remove from heat and strain the liquid into a medium bowl. Mix in the confectioner's sugar and corn syrup until smooth and creamy. Drizzle onto cooled cakes or cookies and let rest for 1 hour before serving.

ROYAL ICING

YIELD: 2 CUPS

This icing has numerous uses, from piping intricate decorations on cookies, to gluing gingerbread houses together. Make this icing right before using for easiest application. For best results, use a piping bag equipped with a small round tip.

2 cups confectioners sugar
3 tablespoons non dairy milk
1 tablespoon corn syrup

- Place all ingredients into a medium bowl and whisk together until very smooth. Use immediately.

RAINBOW SPRINKLES

YIELD: 2 CUPS

DIY sprinkles for cakes and cookies are very simple, and it gives you the option to make your own sprinkles using all-natural food dyes.

1 recipe Royal Icing
4 or 5 different colors of food coloring, paste, or drops

- Prepare the Royal Icing according to recipe directions and divide evenly among four or five small mixing bowls. Place 1 or 2 drops of each color into the individual bowls until the desired colors are achieved. Place one color of icing into a piping bag fitted with a very small round tip (or you can use a plastic storage bag with just the tip of one corner cut off). Pipe a long skinny stream of icing onto a silicone mat or sheet of waxed paper. Repeat with all colors and let dry completely. Once dried, use a sharp knife to cut into small jimmies.

DARK CHOCOLATE GANACHE

YIELD: 2 CUPS

This delicious cake topper couldn't be easier to make, and it only contains two ingredients. Use the best-quality chocolate you can get your hands on for exceptional flavor. Ganache makes a lovely filling in between cakes and cookies, too, especially the Vanilla Wafers.

¾ cup full-fat coconut milk
1½ cups non dairy chocolate chips

• Heat the coconut milk in a small saucepan over medium heat just until it begins to bubble. Remove from heat. Place chocolate chips in small bowl and then stir in hot coconut milk to melt the chips. Let cool until slightly thickened.

73

DEVILISHLY DARK CHOCOLATE SAUCE

YIELD: 1 CUP

Espresso and cocoa powders combine for a sinfully rich sauce. Easy to make, it is great served warm over ice cream, or drizzled onto cheesecakes for an extra-special touch.

⅔ cup dark cocoa powder
½ teaspoon espresso powder
1⅔ cups sugar
1¼ cups water
1½ teaspoons vanilla extract

- In a medium saucepan, whisk together the cocoa powder, espresso powder, sugar, and water. Over medium heat, bring the mixture to a boil and let cook for 1 minute, while stirring constantly. Remove from heat and stir in vanilla extract. Let cool before transferring to an airtight container. Store in refrigerator for up to 2 weeks and reheat to serve warm or use cold.

HOT FUDGE SAUCE

YIELD: 1½ CUPS

Better than the kind you can buy from the store, this hot fudge sauce keeps for up to 1 month if stored in an airtight container in the fridge.

1 cup sugar
⅓ cup cocoa powder
2 tablespoons brown rice flour (superfine is best)
2 tablespoons coconut oil
1 cup non dairy milk
1 teaspoon vanilla extract

- In a small saucepan, whisk together all of the ingredients and heat over medium heat. Continue to stir as the mixture heats, ensuring no lumps remain as the mixture gets hot. Reduce the temperature slightly and continue to cook until thickened, for about 3 to 4 minutes. Stir well right before serving and enjoy hot.

- Store in airtight container in the refrigerator for up to 1 month, and reheat as needed to top ice cream and other goodies.

BUTTERSCOTCH SAUCE

YIELD: 2 CUPS

Salty and sweet butterscotch sauce was always my favorite topper for ice cream. I like having a jar stowed away in the fridge for those inevitable ice cream sundae cravings.

¼ cup non dairy margarine
1 cup packed brown sugar
¾ cup canned full-fat coconut milk
½ teaspoon vanilla extract

- Place the margarine into a 2-quart saucepan over medium heat and melt slightly. Add in the brown sugar and heat until the margarine and sugar have mostly melted.

- Once liquefied, add the coconut milk and vanilla extract and stir well. Continue to cook over medium heat for 9 minutes, stirring often. Turn off heat and let cool slightly. Whisk together well and transfer to a glass jar. Let cool completely before capping and transferring to the refrigerator. This will keep for up to 3 weeks.

CARAMEL SAUCE

YIELD: 1 CUP

This easy caramel sauce was created for topping the Caramel Chai Cheesecake but is also incredible over ice cream, especially with sprinkles.

1 cup brown sugar, packed
½ cup non dairy margarine
¼ cup almond or coconut milk
1¼ teaspoons vanilla extract

- In a 2-quart saucepan, whisk together the ingredients and warm over medium heat. Cook, stirring, just until the mixture has thickened to a creamy caramel sauce consistency, for about 5 minutes. Store in airtight container in refrigerator for up to 2 weeks.

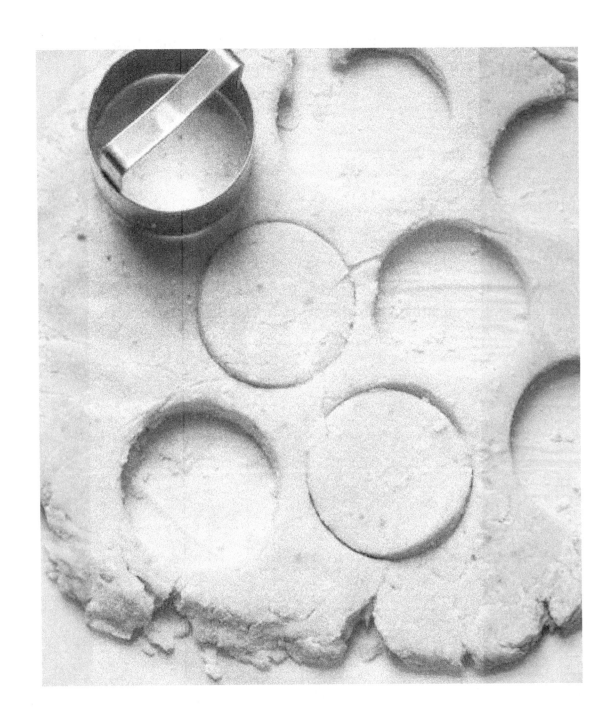

Chapter 3

CAPTIVATING COOKIES AND BARS

Who doesn't love a cookie? They come in all shapes, sizes, textures, flavors, and colors, are easy to prepare, and are always a crowd-pleaser—especially when they are free of a few common allergens, like dairy, eggs, and gluten!

You may want to invest in a few cookie jars to house all these cookies and bars. If the baking bug hits you hard, cookies do make wonderful gifts.

DROP COOKIES

CLASSIC CHOCOLATE CHIP COOKIES

YIELD: 24 COOKIES

Crispy, chewy, and crunchy, these chocolate chippers are just like the ones the corner cookie shop makes. Be sure to let these rest for at least 30 minutes before transferring from cookie sheet.

2 tablespoons flaxseed meal

4 tablespoons water

1 cup non dairy margarine

1 cup sugar

1 cup packed brown sugar

1 teaspoon vanilla extract

1 teaspoon baking soda

2 teaspoons warm water

2 cups sorghum flour

1 cup brown rice flour

½ cup tapioca flour

1 teaspoon xanthan gum

1 cup semi-sweet non dairy chocolate chips

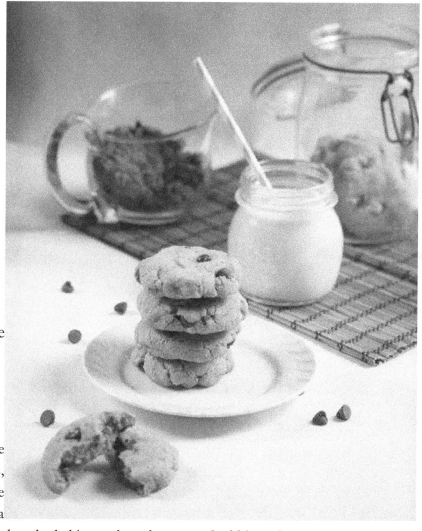

* Preheat oven to 375°F.

* In a small bowl, mix the flaxseed meal with the water and allow it to rest for at least 5 minutes, or until thick. Cream together the margarine and sugars until smooth. Add in the vanilla extract and prepared flaxseed meal. Blend together the baking soda and water and add into the creamed margarine mixture.

* In a separate bowl, whisk together the rest of the ingredients up to the chocolate chips. Gradually stir the flours into the margarine mixture until a clumpy dough forms. It should be doughy, but not sticky. If it is too sticky, you will need to add more sorghum flour, about 1 tablespoon at a time, until it becomes a soft dough.

* Shape the dough into rounded spoonfuls and place onto an ungreased cookie sheet about 2 inches apart. Bake on the middle rack about 11 minutes, or until slightly golden brown on edges.

* Store in airtight container up to 1 week.

OATMEAL RAISIN COOKIES

YIELD: 24 COOKIES

Addictively easy, these are always a welcome addition to a standard cookie tray. If you're like I was as a kid, feel free to sub in chocolate chips for the raisins.

2 tablespoons flaxseed meal
¼ cup water
1 cup non dairy margarine
1 cup brown sugar
1 teaspoon vanilla extract
1 cup brown rice flour
½ cup potato starch
¼ cup tapioca flour
1 teaspoon xanthan gum
1 teaspoon baking powder
3 cups certified gluten-free oats
1 cup raisins

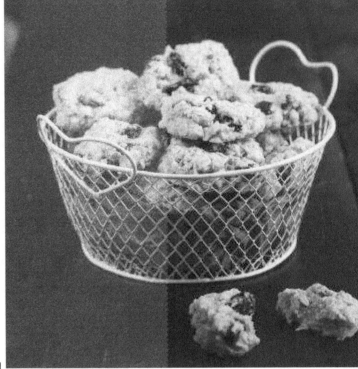

- Preheat oven to 350°F. In a small bowl, combine the flaxseed meal with the water and let rest for 5 minutes, until gelled.

- In a large mixing bowl, cream together the margarine and sugar until smooth. Add in the vanilla extract and the prepared flaxseed.

- In a medium bowl, whisk together the brown rice flour, potato starch, tapioca flour, xanthan gum, and baking powder. Stir into the creamed sugar mixture. Fold in the oats and raisins.

- Shape the dough into about 1½-inch balls and place onto an ungreased cookie sheet about 2 inches apart. Flatten slightly and bake on middle rack for 15 minutes. Let cool completely before serving. Store in airtight container for up to 1 week.

PRETENTIOUSLY PERFECT PEANUT BUTTER COOKIES

YIELD: 24 COOKIES

To be able to call oneself "perfect" takes a good bit of gusto, but man oh man, do these cookies deliver! Chewy, but crunchy, and baked until gloriously golden, these can also be perfect almond, cashew, or sunflower butter cookies if you have a peanut allergy. Simply swap in another nut or seed butter.

½ cup non dairy margarine
¾ cup smooth peanut butter
½ cup sugar
½ cup packed light brown sugar
1 tablespoon flaxseed meal
2 tablespoons water
¾ cup sorghum flour
¼ cup tapioca flour
½ cup potato starch
¾ teaspoon xanthan gum
¾ teaspoon baking soda

- Preheat oven to 375°F.

- In a large mixing bowl, cream together the margarine, peanut butter, and sugars until smooth. In a small bowl, mix the flaxseed meal with the water and allow it to rest for at least 5 minutes, or until thick. Add into the peanut butter mixture.

- In a separate bowl, whisk together the rest of the ingredients and then gradually incorporate into the peanut butter mixture until all has been added and a clumpy dough forms. Roll dough into 1-inch balls and flatten the cookies using a fork, forming a crisscross pattern and pressing down gently but firmly. Place 2 inches apart onto an ungreased cookie sheet.

- Bake for 11 minutes. Remove from the oven but let remain on cookie sheet until completely cooled. Store in airtight container for up to 2 weeks. These also freeze nicely.

SNICKERDOODLES

YIELD: 24 COOKIES

Some speculate that Snickerdoodles have German roots, while others believe that the name "Snickerdoodle" was just another whimsical cookie name made in the nineteenth-century New England tradition. Regardless of the source of the name, these cookies are another childhood favorite.

2 tablespoons flaxseed meal

4 tablespoons water

½ cup non dairy margarine

½ cup non hydrogenated shortening

1½ cups sugar, plus 4 tablespoons for rolling

1 teaspoon vanilla extract

2 teaspoons cream of tartar

2 teaspoons baking soda

½ teaspoon salt

1 cup sorghum flour

1 cup millet flour

¾ cup potato starch

1 teaspoon xanthan gum

1 tablespoon cinnamon, for rolling

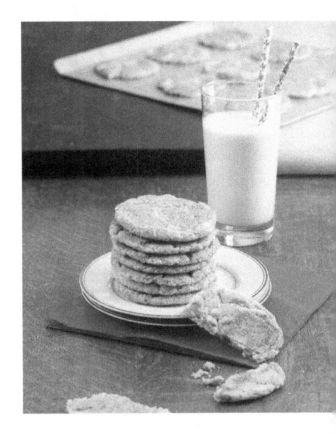

- Preheat oven to 375°F.

- In a small bowl, mix the flaxseed meal with the water and allow it to rest for at least 5 minutes, or until thick.

- Cream together the margarine, shortening, and 1½ cups sugar until smooth. Mix in the prepared flaxseed meal, vanilla extract, cream of tartar, baking soda, and salt.

- In a separate bowl, combine sorghum flour, millet flour, potato starch, and xanthan gum. Slowly combine the flour mixture with the sugar mixture and mix vigorously (or use an electric mixer set on medium-low speed) until a stiff dough forms.

- In another small bowl combine the 4 tablespoons sugar with the cinnamon.

- Roll dough into 1-inch balls and then roll each dough-ball into the cinnamon sugar mixture.

- Place 2 inches apart on an ungreased cookie sheet and bake for 9 minutes.

- Remove from oven, sprinkle with a touch more sugar, and let cool on cookie sheet for about 5 minutes.

- Transfer the cookies to a wire rack and let cool for at least 20 more minutes before handling. Store in airtight container for up to 1 week.

These tender cinnamon sugar–speckled cookies need a lot of space when baking. Be sure to place them at least 2 inches apart on a cookie sheet or the cookies will merge together.

TRAIL MIX COOKIES

YIELD: 24 COOKIES

These cookies feature all my favorite flavors of trail mix baked right into a scrumptious cookie. The options for mix-ins are endless. Try pepitas, dried blueberries, or even your favorite spice blend to shake things up!

½ cup smooth peanut butter
½ cup non dairy margarine
1½ cups turbinado sugar
1 teaspoon vanilla extract
3 tablespoons flaxseed meal
6 tablespoons water
¼ teaspoon salt
1 cup sorghum flour
½ cup brown rice flour
¼ cup almond meal
½ cup potato starch
¼ cup tapioca flour
1 teaspoon xanthan gum
1 teaspoon baking powder
½ cup shredded coconut (sweetened)
1 cup non dairy chocolate chips
½ cup sliced almonds
½ cup raisins

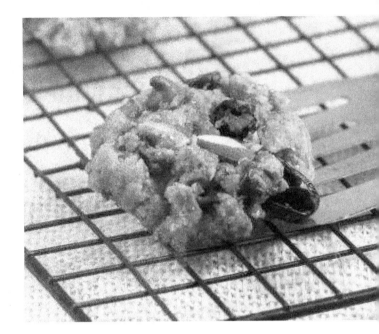

- Preheat oven to 375°F. In a large bowl, cream together the peanut butter, margarine, sugar, and vanilla extract until smooth. In a small bowl, mix the flaxseed meal with the water and allow it to rest for at least 5 minutes, or until thick. Add in the prepared flaxseed meal.

- In a separate bowl, whisk together the salt, sorghum flour, brown rice flour, almond meal, potato starch, tapioca flour, xanthan gum, and baking powder. Gradually add the flour mixture into the peanut butter mixture and mix until a dough forms.

- Fold in the coconut, chocolate chips, almonds, and raisins until incorporated.

- Drop by rounded tablespoonfuls onto an ungreased cookie sheet 2 inches apart. Flatten slightly with the back of a spoon and bake for 12 minutes, or until bottoms are golden brown. Let cool completely on the rack before enjoying. Store in airtight container for up to 1 week.

If you use a sugar other than turbinado, you may need to add 1 to 2 tablespoons of nondairy milk to get a proper dough to form.

SUPER-SOFT CHOCOLATE CHIP PUMPKIN COOKIES

YIELD: 20 COOKIES

Just as the name implies, these cookies are super soft and chock-full of pumpkin goodness. I love making these for Halloween parties, as they are always quick to get gobbled up!

½ cup non dairy margarine

1⅓ cups sugar

1¼ cups canned (or fresh, drained well in cheesecloth) pumpkin puree

1 teaspoon vanilla extract

1 teaspoon baking powder

½ teaspoon baking soda

1 teaspoon sea salt

1¼ cups sorghum flour

¾ cup brown rice flour

½ cup potato starch

¼ cup tapioca flour

1 teaspoon xanthan gum

1 cup non dairy chocolate chips

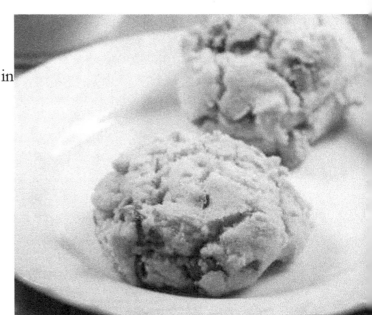

- Preheat oven to 350°F.

- Cream together the margarine and sugar. Once smooth, mix in the pumpkin.

- In separate bowl, mix together the rest of the ingredients except for the chocolate chips. Slowly fold the flour mixture into the pumpkin mixture just until mixed. Fold in the chocolate chips.

- Drop by tablespoonfuls onto an ungreased cookie sheet about 2 inches apart. Bake for 17 minutes. Remove from oven and let cool completely before enjoying. Store in airtight container for up to 1 week.

If using fresh pumpkin with these, be sure to strain the pump kin very well so that very little liquid remains before adding to the cookies.

GARAM MASALA COOKIES

YIELD: 18 COOKIES

If you think garam masala is only good for savory dishes, these cookies will open your eyes! With warming notes of brown sugar, vanilla, and the delicious Indian spice blend, what's not to love?

1 cup cold non dairy margarine

¾ cup sugar

¾ cup brown sugar

1 teaspoon vanilla extract

2 teaspoons baking powder

2 teaspoons garam masala

1 teaspoon xanthan gum

2 tablespoons apple cider vinegar

¼ cup almond flour

1 cup buckwheat flour

½ cup sweet white rice flour

2 tablespoons cocoa powder, for dusting

• Preheat oven to 375°F. Cream together the margarine and sugars. Add the vanilla extract, baking powder, garam masala, and xanthan gum. Add the vinegar and then gradually mix in all of the flours a little at a time until well blended.

• Using a tablespoon, scoop out round balls onto an ungreased cookie sheet about 3 inches apart. Bake for about 10 minutes, or until the cookies have flattened out completely.

• While they are still warm, sprinkle a touch of cocoa powder on each cookie. Store in airtight container for up to 1 week.

MAPLE COOKIES

YIELD: 24 COOKIES

Crispy on the inside and cakey in the middle, these irresistible cookies will have you reaching in the cookie jar again and again with their seductive maple flavor. For an extra-indulgent treat, top with the glaze from Mini Maple Donuts.

1 tablespoon flaxseed meal

2 tablespoons water

½ cup non dairy margarine

½ cup brown sugar

½ cup maple syrup

1 teaspoon maple extract

1 teaspoon baking soda

1¾ cups superfine brown rice flour

1 cup potato starch

¼ cup cornstarch

¼ cup tapioca flour

1 teaspoon xanthan gum

½ teaspoon salt

½ cup turbinado sugar

- Preheat oven to 350°F. Line a cookie sheet with parchment paper. Mix the flaxseed meal with the water in a very small bowl. Let rest for 5 minutes, or until gelled.

- In a large mixing bowl, cream together the margarine, sugar, and maple syrup until fluffy. Mix in the prepared flaxseed meal and maple extract.

- In a medium bowl, whisk together the remaining ingredients, except for the turbinado sugar, and then gradually incorporate into the creamed margarine until a soft dough is formed. Do not overmix.

- Form into 1-inch balls and roll in the turbinado. Flatten slightly with the back of a fork and bake for 15 minutes, rotating the cookie tray after 10 minutes' baking time. Let cool completely before removing from cookie sheet. Store in airtight container up to 1 week.

PECAN SANDIES

YIELD: 24 COOKIES

Be sure to serve with a tall cold glass of almond or rice milk!

1 tablespoon flaxseed meal
2 tablespoons water
½ cup non dairy margarine
½ cup olive oil
½ cup confectioners sugar
½ cup sugar
1¼ cups brown rice flour
½ cup potato starch
¼ cup tapioca flour
1 teaspoon xanthan gum
½ teaspoon baking soda
½ teaspoon cream of tartar
½ teaspoon salt
1 cup chopped pecans, plus 24 whole pecans for topping

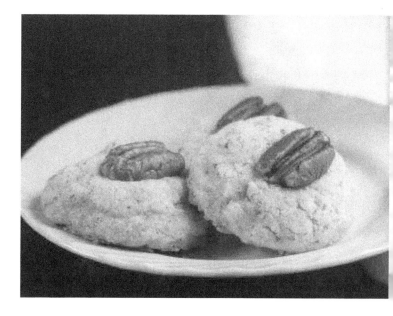

- Preheat oven to 375°F.

- Mix the flaxseed meal with the water in a very small bowl. Let rest for 5 minutes, or until gelled. In a large bowl, mix together the margarine, oil, sugars, and prepared flaxseed meal until blended.

- In a separate bowl, whisk together the brown rice flour, potato starch, tapioca flour, xanthan gum, baking soda, cream of tartar, and salt. Add the flour mixture to the sugar mixture and stir well to combine into a slightly oily dough. Add the chopped pecans.

- Form into 1-inch balls, place 2 inches apart onto an ungreased cookie sheet, and place a single pecan on top of each cookie. Bake for 11 minutes, or until lightly golden on the edges.

- Let cool completely before serving. Store in airtight container for up to 1 week.

COCOA MACAROONS

YIELD: 24 COOKIES

These simple cookies are ooey, gooey, and chewy with a crispy crunchy outer shell. Perfect for snacking. If you want to change it up a bit, try the Australian method and place a small bit of jam or a fruit—such as a dried cherry—inside the coconut dough before baking.

3 tablespoons flaxseed meal
¼ cup + 2 tablespoons water
4 cups sweetened shredded coconut
¼ cup cocoa powder
½ cup sugar
½ teaspoon salt

- Preheat oven to 350°F and line a cookie sheet with a silicone mat or parchment paper.

- In a small bowl, whisk together the flaxseed meal and water and let set for 5 minutes, until gelled. In a medium bowl, stir together the remaining ingredients until blended. Fold in the prepared flaxseed meal and stir well until completely incorporated. The batter will be slightly tricky to squeeze together but will hold well once baked. Drop by tablespoons onto the prepared cookie sheet and bake for 15 to 18 minutes, until fragrant and slightly darkened.

- Let rest for at least 1 hour before serving.

FLORENTINES

YIELD: 12 COOKIES

Even though the name sounds wholly Italian, these cookies most likely originated in French kitchens, with the name simply a nod to the Tuscan city. As beautiful as they are tasty, don't be intimidated by the Florentine; they are a snap to make. Be sure to leave extra space in between each cookie, as they spread! Aim for about six per standard-size cookie sheet.

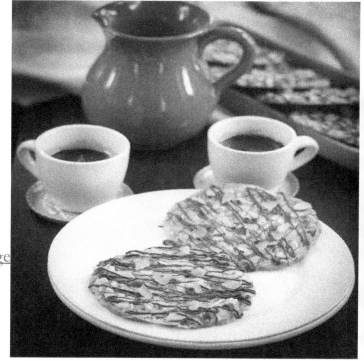

1¼ cups sliced almonds

¼ cup superfine brown rice flour

⅓ cup sugar

4 tablespoons non dairy margarine

¼ cup agave

¼ teaspoon salt

⅓ cup non dairy chocolate, melted

2 tablespoons finely chopped Candied Orange Peels or orange zest

- Preheat oven to 350°F.

- In a medium bowl, combine the almonds and the brown rice flour. In a small saucepan, mix together the sugar, margarine, agave, and salt and bring to a boil, stirring often. Remove immediately from heat and stir mixture into the almond mixture. Mix until totally combined and drop by heaping tablespoons onto a parchment-lined cookie sheet, about 3 inches apart. Using a lightly greased fork, press down cookies into a flat circle, so that the almonds are in a single layer.

- Bake for 5 minutes, rotate the cookie sheet, and bake for 4 to 5 minutes more, until the edges of the cookies are golden brown. Let cool completely and then drizzle with melted chocolate and sprinkle with orange peel. Let chocolate firm up before serving. Store in airtight container for up to 1 week.

THUMBPRINT COOKIES

YIELD: 24 COOKIES

A lovely cookie that is simple to make and easy on the eyes. Sprinkle with confectioners sugar once cooled for an elegant presentation. This cookie works best with low-sugar preserves (my favorites are apricot and raspberry!) or a high-pectin jam. Other types of jams can cause the filling to spread.

1 tablespoon flaxseed meal
2 tablespoons water
1 cup non dairy margarine
1 cup sugar
1 teaspoon vanilla extract
1 teaspoon baking powder
1 cup sorghum flour
1 cup potato starch
1 cup almond meal
1 teaspoon xanthan gum
⅓ cup preserves (1 teaspoon per cookie)

- Preheat oven to 350°F.

- Mix the flaxseed meal with the water in a very small bowl. Let rest for 5 minutes, or until gelled. Line a cookie sheet with parchment paper or a silicone baking mat.

- Cream together the margarine and sugar until smooth. Add in the prepared flaxseed meal and vanilla extract and mix well.

- In a separate bowl, combine the baking powder, sorghum flour, potato starch, almond meal, and xanthan gum.

- Gradually add the flour mixture into the sugar mixture until a stiff dough forms.

- Shape into 1-inch balls and place onto cookie sheet. Use the back of a ½ teaspoon (or your thumb) to make an indent in the cookies while slightly flattening them.

- Fill each cookie with a little less than a teaspoon of preserves. Bake for 15 minutes in preheated oven and then let cool completely. Store in airtight container for up to 4 days.

MEXICAN WEDDING COOKIES

YIELD: 15 COOKIES

These delicately crunchy cookies practically melt in your mouth. Also known as Russian Tea Cakes or Polvorones, it doesn't matter what name you use— once you try them, you'll never forget them.

¾ cup non dairy margarine

½ cup confectioner's sugar, plus ¼ cup for rolling

½ teaspoon salt

1 cup almond meal

1½ teaspoons vanilla extract

¾ cup sorghum flour

½ cup potato starch

¼ cup tapioca flour

1 teaspoon xanthan gum

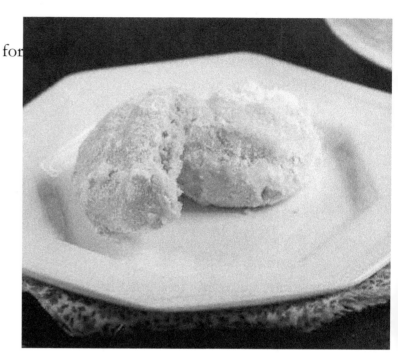

- Preheat oven to 325°F.

- In a large mixing bowl, cream together the margarine and ½ cup confectioner's sugar until smooth. Add the salt, almond meal, and vanilla extract and mix well. In a separate bowl, whisk together the sorghum flour, potato starch, tapioca flour, and xanthan gum.

- Gradually incorporate the flour mixture into the margarine mixture until a clumpy dough forms. Shape into 1-inch balls and place onto an ungreased cookie sheet.

- Bake for 17 to 20 minutes in a preheated oven. Let cool for 2 to 3 minutes, then coat the entire cookie with the additional confectioner's sugar. Let cool completely before serving. Store in airtight container for up to 2 weeks.

CRANBERRY WHITE CHOCOLATE ORANGE CLUSTERS

YIELD: 24 COOKIES

These soft clusters of fragrant citrus, tangy cranberry, and creamy white chocolate will have you reaching in the cookie jar again and again!

2 tablespoons flaxseed meal
4 tablespoons water
½ cup non dairy margarine
½ cup unsweetened applesauce
1 cup sugar
1 teaspoon vanilla extract
½ teaspoon orange zest
1 teaspoon salt
1 teaspoon baking soda
1½ cups superfine or regular brown rice flour
1 cup cornstarch
½ cup tapioca flour
1 teaspoon xanthan gum
½ cup dried cranberries
½ cup non dairy white chocolate chips

- Preheat oven to 375°F.

- In a small bowl, mix together the flaxseed meal and the water and let rest until gelled, for about 5 minutes.

- In a large mixing bowl, cream together the margarine, applesauce, sugar, vanilla extract, and orange zest until smooth. In a medium bowl, whisk together the salt, baking soda, brown rice flour, cornstarch, tapioca flour, and xanthan gum. Gradually incorporate into the sugar mixture until a soft dough forms. Fold in the cranberries and white chocolate chips.

- Drop by the tablespoonful onto a parchment-lined cookie sheet, about 2 inches apart. Bake for 12 to 15 minutes, until golden brown on edges. Let cool completely before serving. Store in airtight container for up to 1 week.

DATE DROP COOKIES

YIELD: 24 COOKIES

Sticky sweet centers are enveloped in a soft cookie to bring you an ultimate treat. My husband, who is admittedly a cookie fanatic, raves about these guys and their irresistible texture. I particularly like them because they are simple to prepare but look so beautiful when baked. For soy-free cookies, use soy- free yogurt.

FILLING

1¼ cup dates, pitted and finely chopped

½ cup water Pinch salt

COOKIES

2 tablespoons ground flaxseed

4 tablespoons water

1 cup non dairy margarine

¾ cup sugar

¾ cup brown sugar

⅓ cup plain unsweetened non dairy yogurt

1 teaspoon vanilla extract

1¼ cups sorghum flour

1 cup superfine brown rice flour

¾ cup cornstarch

¼ cup sweet white rice flour

1 teaspoon xanthan gum

1¼ teaspoons baking soda

½ teaspoon salt

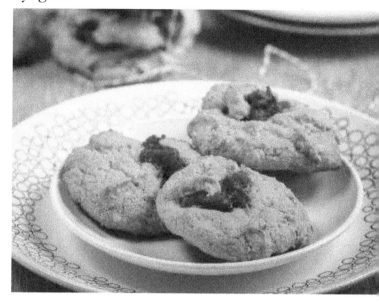

- Place filling ingredients into a 2-quart saucepan and heat over medium heat, stirring often. Cook mixture for 5 minutes, or until thickened. Set aside.

- Preheat oven to 400°F.

- In a small bowl, combine the flaxseed meal with water and allow to gel for 5 minutes, or until thick. In a large mixing bowl, cream together the margarine and sugars until smooth. Add in the prepared flaxseed meal, yogurt, and vanilla extract.

- In a separate bowl, whisk together the rest of the ingredients. Gradually incorporate the flour mixture into the sugar mixture until a clumpy dough forms.

- On an ungreased cookie sheet, drop a tablespoon of the dough. Next, place a teaspoon of the date filling on top of the dough, and then top with a teaspoon more cookie dough. Repeat with all dough and filling. Bake for 11 minutes; let cool completely before serving. Store in airtight container for up to 1 week.

PEANUT BUTTER CHOCOLATE NO-BAKE COOKIES

YIELD: 24 COOKIES

This is one of the very first recipes I learned to make as a kid, and boy did I make them a lot! These were always a favorite due to their quickness and ease and irresistible chocolate peanut butter combo.

¼ cup cocoa powder

2 cups sugar

½ cup almond milk

½ cup non dairy margarine

½ cup + 3 tablespoons creamy peanut butter

1 teaspoon vanilla extract

3½ cups certified gluten-free oats

- Line a large cookie tray with parchment paper.

- In a 2-quart saucepan, combine the cocoa powder, sugar, almond milk, and margarine. Bring to a boil over medium heat, stirring often. Boil for exactly 2 minutes and then remove from heat. Immediately stir in the peanut butter and vanilla extract. Fold in the oats and then drop by spoonfuls on prepared cookie tray. Let rest until firm, for about 1 to 2 hours. Store in airtight container for up to 1 week.

CHERRY COCONUT NO-BAKE COOKIES

YIELD: 24 COOKIES

Tart cherries work so nicely with the base of these no-bakes—perfect for when you're craving cookies, but don't want to turn on the oven.

2 cups sugar

¼ cup coconut oil

2 teaspoons vanilla extract

½ cup non dairy milk

3 cups certified gluten-free oats

⅓ cup dried cherries

½ cup unsweetened flaked coconut

¼ cup almond meal

- Line a large cookie tray with parchment paper.

- In a 2-quart saucepan, over medium heat, combine the sugar, coconut oil, vanilla extract, and nondairy milk. While stirring often, bring the mixture to a boil. Once boiling, continue cooking over medium heat, stirring occasionally, for 1½ to 2 minutes. Remove the mixture from heat and stir in oats, cherries, coconut, and almond meal.

- Drop by heaping tablespoonfuls onto the prepared cookie sheet. While the cookies are still warm, guide them into an evenly round shape using lightly greased fingertips.

- Let the cookies cool for about 1 hour at room temperature. They will harden up nicely.

- Store in airtight container for up to 2 weeks.

BLACK AND WHITE COOKIES

YIELD: 12 COOKIES

If you've never tried a black and white cookie, you are in for a treat. These ginormous lemony beasts boast not one, but two flavors of icing: chocolate *and* vanilla.

½ cup + 1 tablespoon non dairy margarine

¾ cup sugar

½ teaspoon lemon oil or extract

2 teaspoons egg replacer powder (such as Orgran) mixed with 2 tablespoons water

1 cup besan/chickpea flour

½ cup white rice flour

½ cup potato starch

1 teaspoon xanthan gum

½ teaspoon baking powder

¼ teaspoon salt

⅔ cup non dairy milk

1 recipe Chocolate Glaze

1 recipe Vanilla Glaze

- Preheat oven to 350°F. Line a large baking sheet with parchment paper.

- Cream together the margarine and sugar in a large mixing bowl. Add in the lemon oil and prepared egg replacer. In a separate bowl, whisk together the besan, white rice flour, potato starch, xanthan gum, baking powder, and salt. Add it to the margarine mixture and then add in the nondairy milk. Stir well to combine until a fluffy cookie dough is formed. Using an ice cream scoop, drop dough in 3-ounce balls onto the prepared cookie sheet, leaving about 4 inches between each cookie. You will have to make these in multiple batches as they need room to spread.

- Bake for 22 minutes, or until edges are light golden brown. Remove from the oven and let cool completely. Prepare the Vanilla Glaze and frost one half of each of the cookies with the vanilla glaze. Let harden for about 20 minutes, and prepare the Chocolate Glaze. Frost the other half of each cookie with the chocolate glaze. Let harden completely, for about 2 hours, before serving. Store in airtight container for up to 3 days.

GINGER SNAPPERS

YIELD: 24 COOKIES

Crispier than gingerbread, these snappers pack a big ginger flavor into such a small little snack.

1 tablespoon flaxseed meal
2 tablespoons water
1 cup packed light brown sugar
¾ cup olive oil
¼ cup molasses
1 cup sorghum flour
¼ cup superfine brown rice flour
½ cup potato starch
¼ cup tapioca flour
1 teaspoon xanthan gum
2 teaspoons baking soda
1 teaspoon salt
1 teaspoon cinnamon
2 teaspoons fresh grated ginger
½ teaspoon cloves
⅓ cup turbinado sugar, for rolling

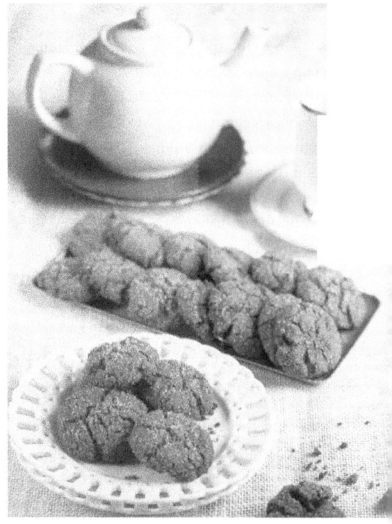

- In a small bowl, combine the flaxseed meal with water and let rest until gelled, for about 5 minutes. Preheat oven to 375°F.

- In a large bowl, mix together the brown sugar, olive oil, molasses, and prepared flaxseed meal.

- In a smaller bowl, whisk together the rest of the ingredients except for the turbinado sugar, and, once mixed, gradually incorporate into the sugar mixture until a stiff dough forms.

- Roll into 1-inch balls and then coat with turbinado sugar. Flatten slightly using the bottom of a glass and bake for 13 minutes in preheated oven. Let cool completely before serving. Store in airtight container for up to 2 weeks.

LEMON OLIVE OIL COOKIES

YIELD: 24 COOKIES

Tender and bright, these cookies are sure to delight! Use freshly squeezed lemon juice and extra-virgin olive oil for best results. If the dough seems a little soft, be sure to chill for about 20 minutes in the refrigerator before baking to prevent excessive spreading.

1 cup sorghum flour
¾ cup brown rice flour
½ cup potato starch
¼ cup almond meal
1 teaspoon xanthan gum
1¼ cups sugar
2 teaspoons baking soda
½ teaspoon salt
2 teaspoons lemon zest
½ cup olive oil
½ cup lemon juice
Granulated sugar for garnishing

- Preheat oven to 350°F.

- In a large bowl, whisk the sorghum flour, brown rice flour, potato starch, almond meal, xanthan gum, sugar, baking soda, and salt. Mix in the lemon zest, olive oil, and lemon juice until a thick cookie dough forms.

- Drop the dough by heaping tablespoonfuls, or roll dough into walnut-size balls and place about 2 inches apart onto an ungreased baking sheet.

- Flatten slightly with a fork (like you would with a peanut butter cookie) and sprinkle lightly with granulated sugar.

- Bake in your preheated oven for 12 minutes, or until edges are slightly golden brown.

- Remove from oven and let cool completely before serving. Store in airtight container for up to 1 week.

ROLLED AND SHAPED COOKIES

VANILLA WAFERS

YIELD: ABOUT 36 COOKIES

A vanilla wafer is always a good cookie to have around for basic reasons, like making into cookie crumbs, using in trifles, and simply snacking. Use the highest-quality vanilla extract you can get your hands on for these, or better yet, make your own.

1 tablespoon flaxseed meal
2 tablespoons water
5 tablespoons non dairy margarine
1 cup sugar
1 tablespoon vanilla extract
¼ cup non dairy milk
¾ cup sorghum flour
½ cup white rice flour
½ cup potato starch
¼ cup tapioca flour
1 teaspoon xanthan gum
2 teaspoons baking powder
¼ teaspoon salt

- Preheat oven to 350°F and line a cookie sheet with parchment paper.

- In a small bowl, stir together the flaxseed meal and water and let rest until gelled, for about 5 minutes.

- In a separate bowl, cream together the margarine, sugar, and vanilla extract until smooth. Mix in the prepared flaxseed meal and nondairy milk.

- In a medium bowl, whisk together the remaining ingredients and then combine well with the margarine mixture until a soft dough forms. Place into a large freezer bag and snip off the tip. Pipe out 1-inch circles onto the parchment-covered cookie sheet about 1 inch apart. Bake for about 20 minutes, or until golden brown on edges. Let cool completely before serving. Store in airtight container for up to 2 weeks.

CHOCOLATE WAFERS

YIELD: 36 COOKIES

Just as versatile as their vanilla cousins, these wafers can wear many hats. Sandwich a little Caramel Frosting in between two cookies or add 1 teaspoon mint extract and dip them in melted chocolate for easy thin mints.

¾ cup cold non dairy margarine
1 cup sugar
1 cup sorghum flour
¾ cup cocoa powder
½ cup potato starch
1 teaspoon xanthan gum
¼ teaspoon baking soda
2 tablespoons strong coffee
¼ cup additional cocoa powder

- Preheat oven to 350°F. Line a large cookie sheet with parchment paper or a silicone baking mat.

- In a large bowl, cream together the margarine and sugar until smooth. In a separate bowl, whisk together the sorghum flour, cocoa powder, potato starch, xanthan gum, and baking soda. Fold the dry ingredients into the sugar mixture and mix until crumbly. Add the coffee and mix until a soft dough forms.

- Gradually fold in the ¼ cup cocoa powder and mix just until dough is workable. Chill in freezer for 5 to 10 minutes and then pinch off sections large enough to create 1-inch balls. Place dough balls onto the prepared baking sheet and flatten with the bottom of a glass to about ¼ inch thick. Bake for 16 minutes. Allow to cool completely before serving. Store in airtight container to keep crisp for up to 2 weeks.

SUGAR COOKIES

YIELD: 24 COOKIES

Sometimes a basic sugar cookie is the best dessert! The secret to these cookies is to keep the dough chilled. I like them best rolled to ¼ inch thick, but you can roll them a touch thinner if you prefer a crispier sugar cookie.

¾ cup non dairy margarine

½ cup sugar

½ cup confectioners sugar

3 teaspoons powdered egg replacer + 2 tablespoons hot water, frothed with fork

2 tablespoons apple cider vinegar

1 teaspoon vanilla extract 1 cup sorghum flour

½ cup white rice flour

¾ cup potato starch

½ cup tapioca flour

1 teaspoon xanthan gum

1 teaspoon baking powder

- Cream together the margarine and sugars until smooth. Mix in the prepared egg replacer along with the vinegar and vanilla extract.

- In a separate bowl, whisk together the sorghum flour, white rice flour, potato starch, tapioca flour, xanthan gum, and baking powder. Gradually combine the flour mixture with the margarine mixture until a clumpy dough forms. If the dough seems too sticky to handle, add a little more sorghum flour … it should be easily workable with your hands, yet a little bit sticky. Form into a patty, wrap in plastic wrap, and chill until cold, for about 1 hour in the refrigerator and 15 minutes in the freezer.

- When your dough is chilled, preheat oven to 400°F. Lay countertop or other work area with parchment paper, and using a lightly floured (any kind of flour will do) rolling pin, roll dough anywhere between ⅓ to ½ inch thick. Cut out using your favorite cookie cutters, and use a flat metal spatula to gently lift the cookies and place them onto an ungreased cookie sheet. Repeat until all dough is used. If the dough seems to be getting a little soft and sticks to your pin, rechill until once again workable.

- Bake cookies for 7 to 8 minutes, or until slightly golden brown on edges.

107

Remove from oven and let cool completely before handling. Store in airtight container for up to 1 week.

- Once they have fully cooled, eat as is or cover them with icing! Royal Icing works beautifully here. Pipe a ring around the cookie's exterior and let harden before filling it in with icing. This will ensure an even layer of icing on the tops with no drips.

BUTTERY SHORTBREAD

YIELD: ABOUT 20 COOKIES

Shortbread used to be considered a delicacy and was reserved for special occasions, such as Christmas or weddings. But no need to wait for a holiday, whip some of these cookies up anytime a craving strikes. This simple cookie can be made extra fancy if you bake them in shortbread molds and dip the ends in melted chocolate.

1 tablespoon flaxseed meal

2 tablespoons water

½ cup + 2 tablespoons non dairy margarine

½ cup sugar

1 teaspoon vanilla extract

¾ cup sorghum flour

¼ cup brown rice flour

¼ cup tapioca flour

½ cup arrowroot starch

¼ cup sweet white rice flour

1 teaspoon xanthan gum

½ cup non dairy chocolate chips, melted, for dipping (optional)

- In a small bowl, combine the flaxseed meal with water and let rest until gelled, for about 5 minutes. In a large mixing bowl, cream together the margarine and the sugar until smooth. Add in the prepared flaxseed meal and vanilla extract and mix until combined.

- In a separate bowl, whisk together the sorghum flour, brown rice flour, tapioca flour, arrowroot starch, sweet white rice flour, and xanthan gum. Gradually mix into the sugar mixture until a clumpy dough forms. The dough may be crumbly at first, but allow enough mixing time for it to come together.

- Wrap the dough in parchment paper and chill for about 30 minutes in the freezer. The dough should be cold, but workable; if it is too crumbly once removed from the freezer, work it a bit with your hands to soften it up.

- Preheat oven to 350°F.

- Create a disk with the dough and place in between two sheets of plastic wrap and roll out to a ¼ inch thickness. Cut using a bench scraper into 2-inch squares, or use a circle cookie cutter, and place onto an ungreased cookie sheet. Bake for 12 minutes, or until bottoms are slightly golden brown. Let cool completely before removing from cookie sheet. At this point, if desired, the cookies can be dipped in melted chocolate and allowed to set backup on a sheet of waxed paper. Store in airtight container for up to 2 weeks.

CHOCOLATE SHORTBREAD

YIELD: 12 COOKIES

Just like the traditional shortbread, only much more chocolaty. I like to cut these into bars, but feel free to shape them as you desire with metal cookie cutters.

1 cup non dairy margarine
½ cup + 2 tablespoons sugar, plus ¼ cup for rolling
½ cup cocoa powder
¾ cup sorghum flour
¾ cup brown rice flour
½ cup potato starch
1 teaspoon xanthan gum

- Cream together the margarine and ½ cup + 2 tablespoons sugar until smooth. Using an electric mixer, or mixing quickly with a spoon, gradually add the cocoa powder.

- In a separate bowl, combine the sorghum flour, brown rice flour, potato starch, and xanthan gum. Add the flour mixture into the sugar mixture (a little bit at a time) until all is incorporated.

- Keep mixing until a stiff dough forms, scraping down the sides as necessary. It will look crumbly at first, but will come together nicely with a little mixing. Using your hands, pat dough into a disk on a lightly sugared surface and then chill the dough in the refrigerator for 2 to 3 hours.

- When you're ready to bake the cookies, preheat oven to 300°F.

- Use a large knife to cut the dough into even rectangles, about 1 × 4 inches. Using a flat metal spatula, scoop up cookies and place them onto an ungreased cookie sheet. Sprinkle with granulated sugar and then poke a few holes in the tops with a fork. Bake for 30 to 35 minutes. Let cool completely before serving. Store in airtight container for up to 2 weeks.

SPECULOOS

YIELD: 24 COOKIES

These cookies have been a favorite of mine long before I ever knew what a speculoos was. I learned this term from the vegan blogging world but soon realized it had been one of my favorites since childhood, only I knew these spicy treats as "windmill cookies." Feel free to roll these out flat and cut with windmill cutters to share in my nostalgia.

1 tablespoon flaxseed meal
2 tablespoons water
1 cup sorghum flour
¼ cup tapioca flour
¼ cup potato starch
½ cup + 2 tablespoons almond meal
1 teaspoon xanthan gum
1 teaspoon baking powder
1 teaspoon cinnamon
¼ teaspoon cloves
¼ teaspoon nutmeg
¼ teaspoon fresh ground ginger
¼ teaspoon salt
½ cup non dairy margarine
¾ cup packed light brown sugar
Extra sugar for sprinkling (optional)
Sliced almonds for topping

- In a small bowl, combine the flaxseed meal with water and let rest until gelled, for about 5 minutes.

- In a large bowl, whisk together all the flour ingredients (up until the margarine) until well blended. In a separate mixing bowl, cream together the margarine and brown sugar until smooth. Mix in the prepared flaxseed meal until a smooth mixture is formed. Gradually add in the flour mixture and mix for about 45 seconds at medium speed until the dough clumps together. Chill in the freezer for 40 minutes, or until stiff—or alternatively, chill in refrigerator overnight.

- Preheat oven to 350°F.

- Once the dough is chilled, use your hands to roll into 1-inch wide balls and place onto an ungreased cookie sheet. Flatten with the bottom of a glass— slightly damp and dipped in granulated sugar. Top with a few sliced almonds and bake in preheated oven for 15 minutes. Let cool on the cookie sheet before attempting to move. Once cool, transfer to wire rack to fully harden.

- Store in airtight container for up to 5 days.

SPECULOOS BUTTER

YIELD: ABOUT 2 CUPS

This cookie butter has taken over the nation from suppliers such as Trader Joe's popularizing it to the extreme … but I've never found one in stores that is gluten-free! So, I had to make my own, and boy am I glad I did. Try this "butter" on top of cupcakes, more cookies, ice cream, or simply a spoon.

24 Speculoos cookies
3 tablespoons water
½ cup coconut oil, melted

- Place the cookies into a food processor and pulse until very crumbly. Make sure the crumbles are finely chopped. Add in the water, one tablespoon at a time and pulse until well blended. Drizzle in the coconut oil and let blend until very smooth, for about 5 minutes, scraping the sides as needed. Transfer into a jar and store in refrigerator. Keep for up to 2 weeks.

PIZZELLES

YIELD: 18 COOKIES

These cookies are delicious on their own but also make a fabulous accompaniment to ice cream, especially when shaped into waffle cones. To make these cookies into homemade waffle cones you will need a Pizzelle press, which can be sourced from any typical home goods store. When hot to the touch, shape the cookie disks into cones, fit inside a small bowl to make waffle bowls; or, leave them flat for classic pizzelle cookies.

3 tablespoons flaxseed meal
6 tablespoons water
1 cup white rice flour
½ cup potato starch
¼ cup tapioca flour
2 teaspoons baking powder
1 teaspoon xanthan gum
1 teaspoon vanilla extract
1 cup melted non dairy margarine
¼ cup water

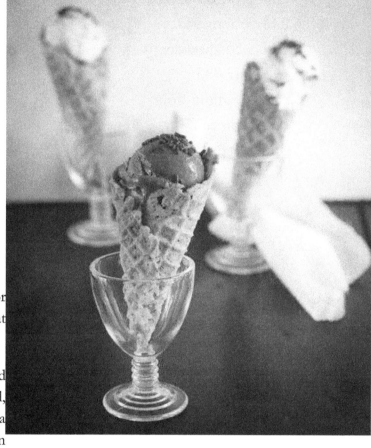

- Preheat the pizzelle press and grease lightly with oil or nonstick spray just before the first batch, and repeat sparingly as needed.

- In a small bowl, mix the flaxseed meal with water and let rest for 5 minutes, until gelled. In a medium bowl, whisk together the rice flour, potato starch, tapioca flour, baking powder, and xanthan gum. Make a well in the center of the flours and add in the vanilla extract, melted margarine, prepared flaxseed meal, and water. Mix until smooth. Place about 1 tablespoon batter onto the hot press and clamp down to close. Cook until golden brown and then gently remove.

- To make waffle cones: Using an oven mitt or heat-safe gloved hands, gently shape the cookie into a cone and snugly place in a safe spot to cool, for about 1 hour. Watch that they don't unravel before cooling or they will become stuck in that shape. Let cool completely, and then serve with your favorite frozen treat. Store in airtight container for up to 3 weeks.

SNOW CAP COOKIES

YIELD: 24 COOKIES

These cookies are a classic right up there next to Chocolate Chip and Peanut Butter. This version includes teff flour, which boasts a pretty impressive nutritional profile for such a tiny grain, being high in protein, iron, calcium, and potassium!

3 tablespoons flaxseed meal

6 tablespoons water

1 cup cocoa powder

½ cup teff flour

¾ cup sorghum flour

¼ cup tapioca flour

½ cup potato starch

1 teaspoon xanthan gum

2 teaspoons baking powder

½ teaspoon salt 2 cups sugar

½ cup melted non hydrogenated shortening

¼ cup non dairy milk

½ cup confectioners sugar

- In a small bowl, combine the flaxseed meal with water and let rest until gelled, for about 5 minutes.

- In a large bowl, whisk together the cocoa powder, teff flour, sorghum flour, tapioca flour, potato starch, xanthan gum, baking powder, salt, and sugar. While stirring constantly, or set on medium speed of an electric mixer, add in the prepared flaxseed meal and shortening until a crumbly dough forms. Mix well to blend. Add in the nondairy milk while continuing to stir and keep mixing until the dough clumps together easily.

- Wrap dough in parchment or foil and chill in refrigerator for 2 hours.

- Once chilled, roll into small balls about 1½ inches wide and flatten slightly to resemble small pucks.

- Preheat oven to 350°F.

- Dip the tops only in confectioner's sugar and place onto an ungreased cookie sheet. Bake for 12 minutes, or until spread out and crackled. The centers will still be gooey while warm. Allow to cool completely before enjoying. Store in airtight container for up to 1 week.

TUXEDO SANDWICH COOKIES
YIELD: ABOUT 20 COOKIES

These cookies taste just like America's favorite sandwich cookie; a touch of orange adds an elegant note. You can even twist off the tops and just enjoy the filling! Dunked in almond milk they become the perfect remedy to the midday slumps.

COOKIES

1 cup non dairy margarine

¾ cup sugar

¼ cup brown sugar

1 teaspoon vanilla extract

¾ cup dark cocoa powder

½ cup superfine brown rice flour

1 cup sorghum flour

½ cup potato starch

1½ teaspoons xanthan gum

1 teaspoon salt

1 teaspoon baking powder

½ teaspoon baking soda

FILLING

1½ tablespoons orange zest

½ cup very cold coconut-based buttery spread (shortening will also work)

½ cup non dairy margarine

3½ cups confectioner's sugar

- Cream together the margarine and sugars and then mix in the vanilla extract. In a separate bowl, whisk together the cocoa powder, superfine brown rice flour, sorghum flour, potato starch, xanthan gum, salt, baking powder, and baking soda.

- Gradually incorporate the flours with the margarine mixture until a clumpy dark dough is formed. Divide and pat into two disks. Chill in the refrigerator for 2 hours, or briefly in freezer, for about 10 minutes.

- After dough is chilled, preheat oven to 350°F and line two cookie sheets with parchment paper.

- On a flat surface, place each chilled disk of dough between two separate sheets of parchment paper and roll each disk to about ⅛ inch thickness. Using a round 2-inch cookie cutter, cut out circles of dough and transfer onto prepared cookie sheets. Bake for 13 minutes and let cool completely before piping filling in between two of the cookies.

- To make the filling, simply mix together all frosting ingredients using an electric mixer with whisk attachment. Whip until fluffy and then pipe a ring onto one cookie and smoosh down with another until an even layer of frosting is snugly set in the middle. Store in airtight container for up to 1 week.

COCONUT CARAMEL COOKIES

YIELD: 24 COOKIES

Similar to the coconut-topped Girl Scout Cookies that are both chewy and crisp, these brilliant bites utilize Medjool dates to stand in for the caramel, adding a little extra goodness.

COOKIES

1 cup non dairy margarine

1 teaspoon vanilla extract

½ cup sugar

1 cup sorghum flour

¾ cup superfine brown rice flour

¾ cup potato starch

1½ teaspoons xanthan gum

TOPPING

20 Medjool dates, pits removed

4 tablespoons non dairy margarine

1 teaspoon vanilla extract

½ teaspoon sea salt

3 tablespoons water

2 cups toasted coconut shreds

2 cups chopped non dairy chocolate

- Cream together the margarine, vanilla extract, and sugar until smooth. In a separate bowl, mix together sorghum flour, brown rice flour, potato starch, and xanthan gum.

- Using an electric mixer, slowly incorporate flour mixture into the margarine mixture and beat on medium-low speed for about 2 minutes, scraping sides as needed to form a stiff dough. Press dough into a disk and chill in refrigerator for an hour or so, or chill in the freezer for about 30 minutes.

- Preheat oven to 300°F.

- Once dough has chilled, roll out gently onto parchment paper. The warmer the dough becomes the softer it will get. Roll to about ½ inch thick. Using a 1½-inch circular cookie cutter, cut out as many circles as possible, saving the scraps, rechilling and rerolling until no dough remains. Cut the centers of the cookies out using a small circular cookie cutter, or the back of an icing tip.

- Place cookies gently onto a parchment-covered cookie sheet and bake for 30 to 35 minutes, or until very lightly golden on edges. Let cool completely before removing from cookie sheet.

- Put dates, margarine, vanilla extract, sea salt, and water into a food processor and blend until very smooth, scraping down sides often. Stir in the toasted coconut. Transfer the mixture into a piping bag fitted with a very wide tip. Pipe a ring of filling carefully onto the cookies and press gently into place using slightly greased fingers. Place upside down onto a piece of waxed paper or silicone mat.

- In a double boiler, place the chocolate into the bowl and warm over medium-low heat until melted. Brush the tops of the inverted cookies with melted chocolate to completely coat. Let the chocolate harden and then flip the cookies over. Drizzle with stripes of chocolate and let harden again. Store in airtight container for up to 1 week.

LEMON SANDWICH COOKIES

YIELD: 24 COOKIES

These dreamy cookies, with crispy wafers and creamy filling, make a wonderful accompaniment to chamomile or green tea.

COOKIES

1 tablespoon flaxseed meal

2 tablespoons water

1⅓ cups superfine brown rice flour

½ cup sorghum flour

¼ cup tapioca flour

½ cup potato starch

1½ teaspoons xanthan gum

¾ teaspoon baking powder

½ teaspoon salt

1 cup sugar

½ cup non dairy margarine

¼ cup lemon juice

Zest of 1 lemon

FILLING

1 teaspoon lemon zest

1 tablespoon lemon juice

½ cup shortening

½ cup non dairy margarine

3½ cups + 2 tablespoons confectioners sugar

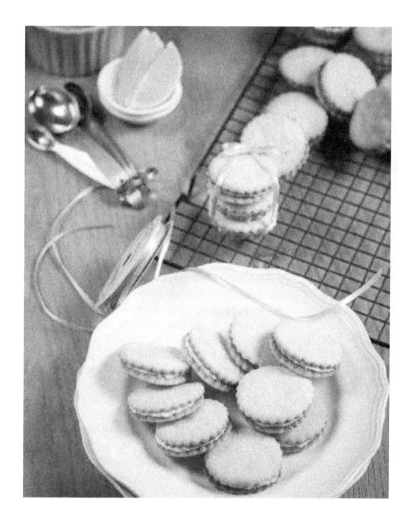

- In a small bowl, combine the flaxseed meal with water and let rest until gelled, for about 5 minutes.

- In a medium bowl, whisk together the superfine brown rice flour, sorghum flour, tapioca flour, potato starch, xanthan gum, baking powder, and salt.

- In a large bowl, cream together the sugar and the margarine until smooth. Add the prepared flaxseed meal, lemon juice, and lemon zest and mix well. Slowly incorporate the flour mixture and stir well until a stiff dough forms. Divide dough into two equal-size disks and chill for at least 1 hour in refrigerator.

- When dough is chilled, preheat oven to 375°F. Roll out one section of dough in between two sheets of parchment paper until about ¼ inch thick. Using a circular cookie cutter, cut out cookies and place onto an ungreased cookie sheet. Repeat until all dough has been used, rechilling the dough if it becomes too soft to work with.

- Bake in preheated oven for 9 minutes. Let cool completely. Make the filling by mixing together all the ingredients in a mixer at high speed until very well combined. Pipe filling onto the back of one cookie and sandwich together with another cookie. Repeat until all cookies have been filled.

- Allow cookies to set for at least 1 hour for best flavor and texture. Store in airtight container for up to 1 week.

ROLLED GINGERBREAD COOKIES

YIELD: 24 COOKIES

Freshly grated ginger really makes these cookies sparkle. Feel free to cut these little guys (or gals) into any shape your heart desires. Roll them thicker for softer cookies, and thinner for crispier.

1 tablespoon flaxseed meal

2 tablespoons water

½ cup non dairy margarine

½ cup sugar

½ cup molasses

1 teaspoon freshly grated ginger

1 teaspoon cinnamon

½ teaspoon nutmeg

½ teaspoon cloves

1¾ cups buckwheat flour, divided

¾ cup potato starch

¼ cup tapioca flour

1 teaspoon xanthan gum

½ teaspoon salt

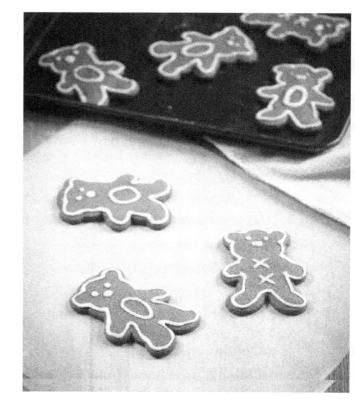

- In a small bowl, stir together the flaxseed meal and water and allow to rest for 5 minutes, until gelled.

- In a large mixing bowl, cream together the margarine, sugar, molasses, ginger, and prepared flaxseed meal. In a separate bowl, whisk together the spices, 1 cup buckwheat flour, potato starch, tapioca flour, xanthan gum, and salt. Add into the sugar mixture and mix until a dough forms. Add up to ¾ cup additional buckwheat flour, until a soft dough that is easy to handle forms. Gently pat the dough into a disk and wrap in parchment paper. Place in freezer and chill for 30 minutes.

- When the dough is chilled, preheat oven to 350°F. Divide dough in half, and roll out one half of dough (while chilling the other half) to about ¼ inch thick. Work fast so the dough stays chilled; the warmer the dough gets, the stickier it becomes. Once rolled, use your favorite cookie cutters to cut out shapes and place the cut cookies directly onto a parchment-covered baking sheet. Bake for 9 minutes. Repeat with the remaining dough and then let cool.

Decorate with Royal Icing. Store in airtight container for up to 2 weeks.

FIGGY FILLED COOKIES

YIELD: 24 COOKIES

These delightful cookies, similar to commercial fig bars, are hearty and not- too-sweet. The key to these cookies is keeping the dough super cold. I advise chilling after each rolling and shaping to ensure stick-free, evenly rolled cookies with no frustration.

COOKIE DOUGH

1½ tablespoons flaxseed meal

3 tablespoons water

⅔ cup cold non dairy margarine

1 cup sugar

1 teaspoon vanilla extract

1⅔ cups brown rice flour

⅔ cup potato starch

⅓ cup tapioca flour

1 teaspoon xanthan gum

2½ teaspoons baking powder

⅓ cup non dairy milk

Additional brown rice flour for rolling

FILLING

2¼ cups dried mission figs, tops removed

¼ cup raisins

1 teaspoon orange zest

1 small apple, diced

½ cup pecans

3 tablespoons sugar

1 teaspoon cinnamon

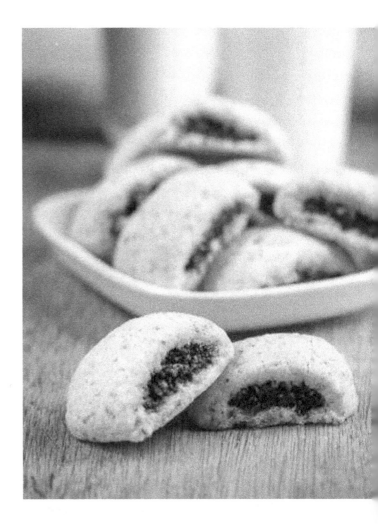

- In a small bowl, combine the flaxseed meal with the water and let rest for about 5 minutes, until gelled.

- In a large mixing bowl, cream together the margarine and sugar until smooth. Mix in the vanilla extract and prepared flaxseed meal.

- In a separate, smaller, bowl, whisk together the brown rice flour, potato starch, tapioca flour, xanthan gum, and baking powder. Gradually add the flour mixture to the sugar mixture and stir well to combine. Add the nondairy milk and mix until a soft dough forms. Dust lightly with brown rice flour if sticky. Wrap in parchment paper and chill in freezer for about 15 minutes, until cold.

- Place all ingredients for the filling into a food processor and pulse until finely crumbled and sticky, scraping down the sides of the bowl as needed.

- Preheat oven to 375°F.

- Take about one-third of the chilled dough and roll it out (in between two sheets of parchment paper) into a rectangle about 3½ inches wide and about
¼ inch thick. Chill briefly, for about 5 minutes in freezer. Roll out a long snake of filling, as you would clay, about 1 inch wide, and place into the center of the rectangle. Fold over each side of the dough, like wrapping a present, using parchment to help roll it up and over, and seal gently using your fingertips. You should have a slightly flat, long enclosed dough tube of figgy filling.

- Chill again briefly, for about 5 minutes. Flip filled dough over to hide the seam on the bottom.

- Using a very clean, sharp, flat blade, cut into 2-inch sections, so that you end up with shapes that look like a popular store-bought variety of fig cookies. Place 2 inches apart onto a parchment-lined cookie sheet. Bake for 15 to 17 minutes or until slightly golden brown on edges. Store in airtight container for up to 1 week.

SPRINGERLES

YIELD: 30 COOKIES

These cookies taste wonderful with or without the use of a Springerle mold, so feel free to let them remain flat on top if you don't have molds handy.

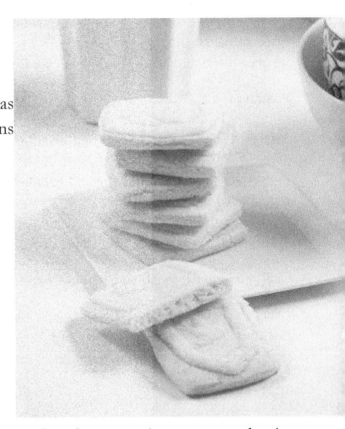

¾ cup non dairy margarine

1 cup sugar

1 teaspoon anise extract

2½ teaspoons powdered egg replacer, such as Orgran or EnerG, mixed with 3 tablespoons water

1 cup superfine brown rice flour

½ cup millet flour

1 cup potato starch

¼ cup tapioca flour

1 teaspoon xanthan gum

1 teaspoon baking powder

½ teaspoon baking soda

¼ teaspoon salt

- Preheat oven to 350°F. In a large bowl, cream together the margarine, sugar, and anise extract. Add the prepared egg replacer.

- In a separate bowl, whisk together the rest of the ingredients. Gradually add into the margarine mixture and mix very well until a clumpy dough forms. Roll dough out to about ½ inch thickness. Lightly dust a Springerle mold with superfine brown rice flour, emboss a pattern into the tops of the dough, and then cut cookies to size with a knife. Carefully transfer onto an ungreased baking sheet. Let rest for 1 hour, and then bake for 15 minutes, until very lightly browned on edges and bottoms. To prevent cracking, prop your oven door open an inch or so while baking. Let cool completely before using a spatula to remove. Store in airtight container for up to 1 week.

CINNAMON GRAHAM CRACKERS

YIELD: 30 CRACKERS

A perfect base for so many recipes, such as s'mores or cheesecake crusts, these crispy crackers are also pretty great on their own. These are especially good slathered with a bit of almond or coconut butter.

1 cup buckwheat flour
1 cup superfine brown rice flour
¼ cup tapioca flour
¾ cup cornstarch
2 teaspoons xanthan gum
1 teaspoon baking powder
½ teaspoon baking soda
1 teaspoon cinnamon
½ cup cold non dairy margarine
½ cup packed brown sugar
1 teaspoon vanilla extract
⅓ cup non dairy milk
¼ cup agave
¼ cup molasses
3 tablespoons turbinado sugar mixed with
½ teaspoon cinnamon

- In a large bowl, whisk together the buckwheat flour, superfine brown rice flour, tapioca flour, cornstarch, xanthan gum, baking powder, baking soda, and cinnamon until thoroughly mixed.

- In a separate bowl, cream together the margarine and sugar until smooth. Mix in the vanilla extract, nondairy milk, agave, and molasses. Gradually add in the flour mixture until all are incorporated and continue to mix until a stiff dough is formed. Add a touch more buckwheat flour if it is sticky.

- Divide into two sections and pat into disks. Preheat oven to 350°F. Chill each disk briefly (about 15 minutes in freezer), and then roll out in between two pieces of parchment paper until a little less than ¼ inch thick. Cut into squares and poke holes in the top (I used the tip of a chopstick) to poke holes and also to perforate the cracker. For easy rolling and transferring, keep the dough cold. If it starts to lose shape easily, pop it back in the freezer (still on the rolling parchment) for a few minutes, and then go back to shaping the crackers.

- The dough will be quite flexible and very easy to pull off the parchment. Use a flat metal spatula to help you if needed. Place onto an ungreased cookie sheet, sprinkle lightly with the mixture of turbinado and cinnamon, and bake in preheated oven for about 12 to 14 minutes, or until firm and a touch darker on edges.

- Let cool completely. Store in airtight container for up to 1 week.

RUGELACH

YIELD: 20 COOKIES

My mother knows how to make some killer rugelach. While it's a traditional Jewish pastry that is enjoyed year-round, the cookies' fragrant fruit filling and crispy pastry crunch always marked the start of the holiday season in our house.

¼ cup soft dried apricots
½ cup dates, not too soft
1¼ cups walnuts
½ teaspoon cinnamon
¼ teaspoon nutmeg
¼ teaspoon salt
¼ cup sugar
1 to 1½ tablespoons apricot or strawberry jam
1 recipe Puff Pastry

- Preheat oven to 400°F. Place the apricots, dates, walnuts, cinnamon, nutmeg, salt, and sugar into a food processor and pulse until well combined. Add in the jam, 1 tablespoon at a time until the mixture clumps together.

- Roll out one-half of the puff pastry in between two sheets of parchment paper into a 12-inch circle. Using a pizza cutter, cut about ten even triangles. Place a small ball of the filling at the small tip of the triangle. Beginning at the opposite side, roll dough up to cover, sealing the tip when the filling is all bundled up. Repeat with the other half of the dough. Place the cookies onto an ungreased cookie sheet on the middle rack of the oven, about 1 inch apart, and bake for 20 minutes, or until golden brown. Store in airtight container for up to 2 weeks.

CRISPY GLAZED LIME COOKIES
YIELD: ABOUT 12 COOKIES

These zingy cookies are delicious on their own and make an exceptional treat served with a scoop of Strawberry Ice Cream. Or, cut them slightly larger, then stuff with your favorite ice cream and freeze for an irresistibly sweet and tangy treat.

COOKIES

¾ cup cold shortening

⅓ cup powdered confectioners sugar

¼ cup sugar

Zest of 1 lime (about 1 teaspoon)

2 tablespoons lime juice

½ teaspoon salt

1¼ cups sorghum flour

½ cup arrowroot starch

¼ cup tapioca flour

1 teaspoon xanthan gum

GLAZE

1 cup confectioners sugar

5 tablespoons freshly squeezed lime juice

Lime zest to garnish

• Cream together the shortening, sugars, lime zest, and lime juice until smooth. In a separate bowl, whisk together the salt, sorghum flour, arrowroot starch, tapioca flour, and xanthan gum and then gradually incorporate into the sugar mixture while mixing just until a firm dough is formed. Flatten into a disk and chill in the freezer for about 15 minutes. While the dough chills, preheat oven to 350°F.

• Roll out dough in between two sheets of plastic cling wrap onto a flat surface until about ¼ inch thick. Cut into 2-inch squares and place onto an ungreased cookie sheet.

• Bake for 15 minutes. Let cool and add glaze to the tops. To make the glaze, simply whisk together the glaze ingredients until completely smooth and runny. Spoon onto the tops of the cookies and let dry about 10 minutes. Spoon on another layer and top with lime zest. Let glaze completely harden before serving. Store in airtight container for up to 1 week.

PALMIERS

YIELD: 18 COOKIES

These prim and proper cookies are sure to impress at your next gathering with friends. They are so elegant and gorgeous, you won't believe how easy they are if you already have puff pastry on hand.

1 recipe Puff Pastry
1 cup turbinado sugar
1 tablespoon cornstarch mixed with 3 tablespoons water

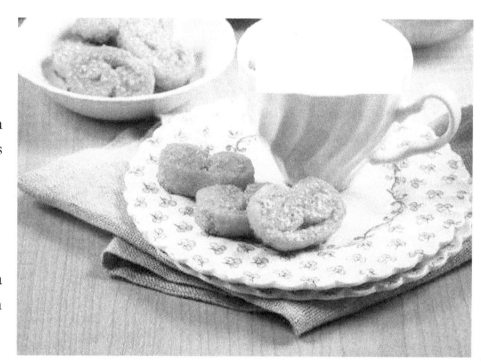

- Preheat oven to 450°F. Line a large baking sheet with parchment paper.

- Divide the puff pastry in two sections and roll each out into two rectangles, about 12 inches by 6 inches. Dust the tops of each rectangle with ½ cup turbinado sugar to evenly cover. Starting from the edges of the two longest sides of the rectangle, roll the edges of the cookie inward, rolling two separate coils so that they face each other and eventually meet. You will have a long tube with two distinct sections. Cut into ½-inch-wide cookies and place directly onto the prepared cookie sheet. Brush with cornstarch mixture. Sprinkle with additional turbinado. Bake for 12 minutes, or until golden brown. Let cool completely before serving. Store in airtight container for up to 1 week.

LAVENDER ICEBOX COOKIES

YIELD: ABOUT 30 COOKIES

Fresh lavender buds are best for these, but, if you don't have fresh, dried will certainly do. You can source dried lavender either online or in specialty herb stores; look for buds that have a nice deep lavender color on the tips. I like to place dried buds in an airtight glass container with an orange or lemon peel for about 1 hour before using to soften them up a bit.

1¼ cups sorghum flour

½ cup brown rice flour (superfine is best, but either can be used)

½ cup potato starch

¼ cup tapioca flour

1⅓ cups confectioners sugar

1 teaspoon xanthan gum

1 cup very cold non dairy margarine

1 tablespoon flaxseed meal

2 tablespoons water

½ cup granulated sugar for rolling

3 tablespoons fresh or dried lavender buds for rolling

- In a food processor, combine all the ingredients up through the xanthan gum and pulse several times to combine thoroughly. Add in the margarine, about a tablespoon at a time, and continue to pulse until crumbly. In a small bowl, combine flaxseed meal with water and let rest until gelled, for about 5 minutes. Add in the prepared flaxseed meal and mix well until a tacky dough forms.

- Divide dough into two sections and shape each as best you can into a log using two pieces of parchment paper. To make perfectly round logs, freeze each log for about an hour, then roll (while still in the parchment) onto a flat surface to create a more even cylinder. Return to freezer and chill at least an additional hour and up to overnight.

- Once ready to bake, preheat oven to 350°F and spread another piece of parchment or foil with a mixture of the granulated sugar and lavender. On a flat surface, roll the log gently but firmly into the mixture to coat, making sure not to be too rough to break the dough. Slice using a sharp knife into ½-inch-thick rounds and place onto an ungreased cookie sheet.

- Bake for 15 to 17 minutes, or until puffy and bottoms are light golden brown. Let cool completely before eating. Store baked cookies in airtight container for up to 1 week.

MOCHA CRUNCHERS

YIELD: 36 COOKIES

Espresso and chocolate meet for a dark and delightful cookie that is easy to roll out and even easier to indulge in! These cookies freeze well both as a dough or prebaked. Simply thaw at room temperature for 30 minutes before baking or enjoying.

2 tablespoons flaxseed meal

¼ cup water

⅔ cup non hydrogenated shortening

1 cup sugar

1 teaspoon baking soda

1 teaspoon salt

1 teaspoon xanthan gum

1¼ cups brown rice flour

⅓ cup cocoa powder

½ cup teff flour

½ cup tapioca flour

2 teaspoons instant espresso powder

1 tablespoon non dairy milk

⅓ cup non dairy chocolate chips

- Preheat oven to 375°F. In a small bowl, mix the flaxseed meal with the water and allow to rest until gelled, for about 5 minutes.

- In a large mixing bowl, cream together the shortening and sugar along with the prepared flaxseed meal. Mix until smooth.

- In a separate bowl, whisk together the baking soda, salt, xanthan gum, brown rice flour, cocoa powder, teff flour, tapioca flour, and instant espresso powder. Bring together the shortening mixture and flour mixture until a crumbly dough forms and, while still mixing, add in the 1 tablespoon non dairy milk until the dough comes together. Form into two even disks and roll out in between two sheets of parchment paper until ¼ inch thick. Cut out using a cookie cutter and transfer to an ungreased cookie sheet using a flat metal spatula. Bake for 9 minutes. Remove from the oven and sprinkle chocolate chips over the hot cookies. Let set for 1 minute and then spread chocolate thinly over the tops of the cookies. Let cool completely before serving. Store in airtight container for up to 1 week.

MATCHA COOKIES

YIELD: 24 COOKIES

Matcha is the powder of finely milled green tea leaves, most often used as a ceremonial tea. Seek out the highest-quality matcha you can for the best flavor. Matcha can be sourced from tea shops, online, and in many grocery chains that offer specialty items, such as Whole Foods.

1 tablespoon flaxseed meal

2 tablespoons water

¼ cup + 3 tablespoons non dairy margarine

⅓ cup confectioners sugar

2 tablespoons sugar

¾ cup sorghum flour

¼ cup tapioca flour

¼ cup potato starch

⅓ cup + 1 tablespoon almond meal

1 teaspoon xanthan gum

2 tablespoons matcha powder

- In a small bowl, mix together the flaxseed meal and water and let rest until gelled, for about 5 minutes.

- In a separate bowl, cream together the margarine and sugars until smooth. Add in the prepared flaxseed meal.

- In another bowl, whisk together the flours, potato starch, almond meal, xanthan gum, and matcha powder and then combine with the margarine mixture to form a soft, but workable dough. If the dough is too sticky, add a touch more sorghum flour until easy to handle. Wrap in plastic wrap and chill in freezer for about 15 minutes. While the dough chills, preheat oven to 350°F and line a cookie sheet with parchment paper or a silicone mat.

- Roll out the chilled dough to a thickness of ¼ inch in between two sheets of parchment paper. Remove top piece of parchment and cut into desired shapes using cookie cutters. Slide the bottom piece of parchment and the cookies onto a cookie sheet and chill for an additional 5 minutes in the freezer, or 15 minutes in the fridge. Using a flat metal spatula, carefully transfer the cut cookies to a parchment-covered baking sheet. Sprinkle with sugar and bake for 12 minutes. Let cool completely before serving. Store in airtight container for up to 1 week.

Have a matcha latte while the cookies bake! To make a simple latte, simply add 1 teaspoon matcha powder to 1 cup very hot non dairy milk. Froth with fork, add a touch of stevia or agave to taste. Voilà! Matcha bliss.

LADYFINGERS

YIELD: ABOUT 36 LADYFINGERS

Use these as the base for Tiramisu or eat alone. When mixing, be sure to measure exactly as even a little too much liquid can cause these cookies, which are chickpea-based, to spread and become flatter than desired. If you have one available, a nonstick, lightly greased ladyfinger pan comes in handy for baking perfect ladyfingers.

½ cup brown rice flour

½ cup + 3 tablespoons besan/chickpea flour

2 tablespoons tapioca flour

2 tablespoons potato starch

2½ teaspoons baking powder

¼ teaspoon salt

½ teaspoon xanthan gum

¾ cup sugar

1 teaspoon apple cider vinegar

½ cup non dairy margarine, softened

⅔ cup non dairy milk

- Preheat oven to 375°F. Lightly spray a ladyfinger pan with a nonstick cooking spray or line a heavy cookie tray with parchment.

- In a large bowl, whisk together the dry ingredients until well mixed. Add the vinegar, margarine, and nondairy milk and mix vigorously until fluffy. Place into a piping bag fitted with a wide round tip and pipe about 1 tablespoon batter into the ladyfinger pan template or in a straight line, about 2 inches apart, straight onto the parchment paper. Be careful not to pipe too much batter or the cookies will spread.

- Bake for 13 to 15 minutes, or until golden brown on edges. Let cool completely before serving. Store in airtight container for up to 1 week.

MADELEINES

YIELD: 24 COOKIES

These light and crisp cookies are perfect any time you want a treat but want to avoid anything that's overly heavy or dense. You'll want to pick up a madeleine pan or two to make these, but these can easily be sourced for under $10 at most kitchen supply stores or online.

3 teaspoons baking powder

¼ teaspoon salt

½ cup white rice flour

½ cup + 2 tablespoons besan/chickpea flour

2 tablespoons tapioca flour

3 tablespoons potato starch

½ teaspoon xanthan gum

1 cup confectioners sugar

1 teaspoon apple cider vinegar

½ cup non dairy margarine

½ cup non dairy milk

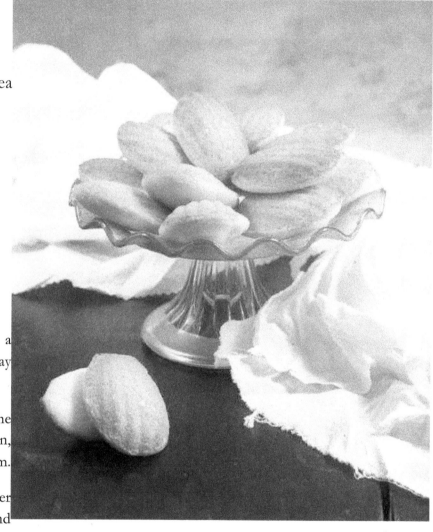

- Preheat oven to 375°F. Lightly spray a madeleine pan with a nonstick cooking spray or grease lightly with olive oil.

- In a large mixing bowl, whisk together the baking powder, salt, white rice flour, besan, tapioca flour, potato starch, and xanthan gum.

- Add the confectioner's sugar, apple cider vinegar, margarine, and nondairy milk and mix on high speed (or very fast using a sturdy balloon whisk) for 2 minutes using a whisk attachment until the batter is fluffy and smooth.

- Spoon about 2 teaspoons of batter into the madeleine molds and spread evenly using a small knife. The cookie molds should be three-quarters full. Rap the pan on an even surface a few times to remove any air pockets.

- Bake for 11 to 13 minutes, or until dark golden brown on seashell side and light blond on the bottoms. Let cool before gently removing from the molds. Store in airtight container for up to 1 week.

HOLIDAY SPRITZ

YIELD: 48 COOKIES

These small, classic holiday cookies can be easy to make, but a little finesse is always appreciated. I recommend a metal cookie press over any others as the dough tends to stick less to them. Also, make sure the dough is chilled before piping for perfect results.

2 teaspoons egg replacer powder (such as Orgran)
2 tablespoons water
1½ cups brown rice flour
½ cup white rice flour
⅔ cup potato starch
1 teaspoon xanthan gum
1 cup non dairy margarine
1 cup confectioners sugar
1½ teaspoons vanilla extract

- In a small bowl, whisk together the egg replacer powder and the water. In a large bowl, whisk together the brown rice flour, white rice flour, potato starch, and xanthan gum. Cream together the margarine, sugar, and vanilla extract and then add the egg replacer mixture. Gradually add the flour mixture until a stiff dough forms. If dough seems too soft, add up to 2 tablespoons brown or white rice flour. Chill for 2 hours in refrigerator, until very cold.

- Preheat oven to 400°F.

- Place in cookie press and fit with disk of choice. Assemble press as instructed and press cookies into desired shapes onto a parchment-covered cookie sheet. Work quickly and be sure to keep the dough cold; this is key! Bake cookies for 7 minutes or until lightly golden brown on edges. Let cool completely before serving. Store in airtight container for up to 3 weeks.

BARS

CHERRY ALMOND BISCOTTI

YIELD: 20 BISCOTTI

This tart and slightly sweet cookie complements tea or coffee beautifully with its fruity notes. Not only is it pleasing to the taste buds, your eyes are in for a treat with deep red cherries studded throughout.

2 tablespoons flaxseed meal
4 tablespoons water
⅓ cup non dairy margarine
¾ cup sugar
1½ teaspoons almond extract
½ teaspoon salt
2 teaspoons baking powder
1 cup sorghum flour

¾ cup brown rice flour
½ cup potato starch
1 teaspoon xanthan gum
¼ cup non dairy milk
1 cup dried cherries

- Preheat oven to 325°F. Combine the flaxseed meal and water into a bowl and let rest for 5 minutes, until gelled.

- In a large bowl, cream together the margarine and sugar until smooth. Add the prepared flaxseed meal, almond extract, and salt.

- In a separate bowl, whisk together the baking powder, sorghum flour, brown rice flour, potato starch, and xanthan gum. Gradually incorporate into the sugar mixture. Add non dairy milk, 1 tablespoon at a time, until a soft dough forms. It should be just dry enough to handle and shape into two balls. Add a touch more sorghum flour or milk to create the right consistency. The dough shouldn't crumble apart, but it also shouldn't be too sticky. Fold in the dried cherries until even distributed.

- Directly on an ungreased cookie sheet, shape the cookie dough into two ovals, about 2.5 inches wide and 1.25 inches tall. Bake in preheated oven for about 30 minutes, until lightly golden on edges. Let cool and then slice cookies diagonally. Place freshly cut cookies on their sides and bake an additional 8 minutes. Turn cookies over and bake another 8 minutes. And one more time … flip, and bake a final 8 minutes. Let cool completely before enjoying. Store in airtight container for up to 3 weeks.

MARBLE BISCOTTI

YIELD: 18 BISCOTTI

Chocolate and vanilla mingle in this delightful-looking cookie. Dip into piping hot coffee or hot chocolate for the ultimate biscotti experience. If you're sharing, these make great gifts once you wrap them up in shiny plastic wrap and adorn them with a bow, especially when paired with your favorite blend of coffee.

3 tablespoons flaxseed meal

6 tablespoons water

½ cup sugar

½ cup non dairy margarine

½ teaspoon vanilla extract

1 cup sorghum flour

¾ cup brown rice flour

½ cup potato starch

¼ cup tapioca flour

1 teaspoon xanthan gum

1½ teaspoons baking powder

½ teaspoon salt

½ cup non dairy chocolate chips, melted, plus 1 cup chocolate chips, melted, for drizzling

- Preheat oven to 325°F.

- In a small bowl, combine flaxseed meal with water and let rest until gelled, for about 5 minutes. In large mixing bowl, cream together the sugar and the margarine. Add the prepared flaxseed meal and vanilla extract and mix well. In a separate bowl, combine the sorghum flour, brown rice flour, potato starch, tapioca flour, xanthan gum, baking powder, and salt. Stir well to evenly incorporate.

- Slowly combine the flour mixture with the margarine mixture until clumpy. Divide dough into two sections, leaving half in the mixing bowl and setting the rest aside. Gently stir in the ½ cup melted chocolate chips with one-half of the dough until very well combined, scraping bowl as needed.

- Now you will have two sections of dough: one chocolate and one vanilla. Shape the vanilla dough into two balls. Shape the chocolate mixture into two balls as well. Then, roll each section into long ropes, so that you have four long ropes of both chocolate and vanilla—about 10 inches long each.

- Working on an ungreased baking sheet, place one chocolate rope and one vanilla rope side by side and then twist over one another, pressing together to form a flat log about 3 inches by 10 inches and then repeat with other two ropes.

- Bake for 28 minutes, until lightly golden brown on edges, and then remove from the oven and place onto a wire rack to let completely cool. Using a serrated knife, slice diagonally into 3 × 1-inch cookies and place freshly cut cookies on their sides on the cookie sheet.

- Bake cookies for 10 minutes. Flip and bake for 10 more minutes. Flip one more time and bake for 5 more minutes. Let cool completely and then drizzle or coat one side with melted chocolate.

- Store in airtight container for up to 1 month.

ULTIMATE FUDGY BROWNIES

YIELD: 12 BROWNIES

These brownies boast a crispy, flaky, paper-thin layer atop a chewy, gooey perfect square of brownie bliss. Even though these brownies are pretty delicious all by their lonesome, they do take kindly to a thin layer of frosting on top, too. Try them topped with Fluffy Chocolate Frosting or Caramel Frosting for an extra- indulgent treat!

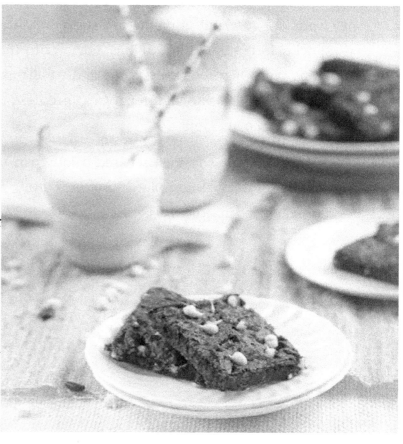

¾ cup superfine brown rice flour

¼ cup almond meal

¼ cup potato starch

¼ cup sorghum flour

1 teaspoon xanthan gum

½ teaspoon baking soda

1 teaspoon salt

3 cups chopped non dairy chocolate or chocolate chips

1 cup sugar

¼ cup non dairy margarine

½ cup strong coffee

2 tablespoons ground chia seed mixed with 5 tablespoons hot water

1 teaspoon vanilla extract

1 cup non dairy white chocolate chips (optional)

- Preheat oven 325°F and lightly grease a 9 × 13-inch metal pan.

- In a large electric mixing bowl, whisk together the superfine brown rice flour, almond meal, potato starch, sorghum flour, xanthan gum, baking soda, and salt.

- Place the chocolate chips into a large heat-safe bowl.

- In a 2-quart saucepan over medium heat, combine the sugar, margarine, and ¼ cup of the coffee and bring to a boil, stirring often. Once boiling, immediately remove from the heat and pour the hot sugar mixture directly onto the chocolate chips, stirring quickly to combine thoroughly. Transfer to the mixing bowl containing the flour mixture along with the prepared chia gel and vanilla extract and mix on medium-high speed until smooth. Add in the additional ¼ cup coffee and mix well. If you're using them, fold in white chocolate chips.

- Spread the batter in the prepared baking pan—the batter will be tacky. Bake for 45 to 50 minutes. Let cool completely before cutting into squares and serving. Store in airtight container for up to 3 days.

BLONDIES

YIELD: 12 BLONDIES

Blondies are lighter than brownies in taste, texture, and color but still bear a delicious resemblance to their chocolate pals. Try these topped with Peanut Butter Banana Ice Cream.

2 tablespoons flaxseed meal
4 tablespoons water
⅓ cup coconut palm sugar
1 teaspoon vanilla extract
1 cup brown rice flour
½ cup almond meal
¼ cup potato starch
1 teaspoon xanthan gum
½ teaspoon salt
½ cup non dairy margarine
1 tablespoon coconut oil
1½ cups non dairy white chocolate chips or pieces
½ cup non dairy mini chocolate chips

- Preheat oven to 350°F. Lightly grease an 8 × 8-inch baking pan.

- In a small bowl, combine the flaxseed meal and water and let rest until gelled, for about 5 minutes. Stir in the coconut palm sugar and vanilla extract. In a separate bowl, whisk together the brown rice flour, almond meal, potato starch, xanthan gum, and salt.

- Over a double boiler, on medium-low heat, melt the margarine, coconut oil, and white chocolate until smooth. Remove from heat. Stir white chocolate mixture into the flour mixture along with the flaxseed meal mixture until a batter forms. Fold in the mini chocolate chips. Press the batter into the prepared baking pan and bake for 27 minutes, or until golden brown on edges. Let cool completely, for at least 2 hours, before serving. Store in airtight container for up to 1 week.

LIGHTEN UP LEMON BARS

YIELD: 16 BARS

These are a lightened-up version of traditional lemon bars, leaving out the eggs and butter and opting for plant-based ingredients instead. Agar can easily be sourced at local health food stores or Asian markets. If you can only source agar bars or flakes, simply run them through a spice grinder until powdered.

CRUST

2 tablespoons flaxseed meal

4 tablespoons water

1½ cups almond meal

¼ teaspoon salt

3 tablespoons sugar

FILLING

2 cups water

1½ tablespoons agar powder

1¼ cups sugar

1 cup freshly squeezed lemon juice (about 6 lemons' worth)

1 drop natural yellow food coloring

¼ cup cornstarch dissolved completely in ¼ cup water

Confectioner's sugar, for dusting

- Preheat oven to 400°F.

- In a small bowl, mix the flaxseed meal with the water until gelled, for about 5 minutes. In a medium bowl, whisk together the rest of the crust ingredients and then massage the prepared flaxseed meal into the almond meal mixture until well blended. Press crust into a lightly greased 8 × 8- inch baking pan. Bake for 12 to 15 minutes, until golden brown on edges. Remove from oven and let cool while you make the filling.

- To make the filling, bring the 2 cups water and agar powder to a boil over medium heat, stirring constantly with a whisk. Let boil for 3 to 5 minutes, until thickened and all agar has dissolved. (Be sure that all agar has dissolved or your lemon bars won't set correctly.) Stir in the sugar, lemon juice, food coloring, and cornstarch slurry. Continue to cook over medium heat, bringing back up to a boil. Let boil for about 3 minutes, until thickened. Pour the mixture on top of the crust and chill immediately on a flat surface in your refrigerator. Chill 2 hours, or until firm. Cut into squares. Dust with confectioners sugar before serving. Store in refrigerator for up to 1 week.

BLUEBERRY BARS

YIELD: 16 BARS

These delicious bars are similar to boxed cereal bars, only tastier and without any added preservatives or chemicals! If blueberry's not your favorite, feel free to use any other type of preserves for endless flavor variations.

1½ cups pecans

1½ cups sorghum flour, plus more as needed for rolling and shaping

⅓ cup potato starch

1 teaspoon baking powder

1 teaspoon xanthan gum

¾ cup non dairy margarine

1 cup sugar

2 tablespoons flaxseed meal

4 tablespoons water

1 cup high-quality blueberry preserves

- Preheat oven to 400°F. Lightly grease and flour the bottom and sides of an 8 × 8-inch baking pan.

- Lay pecans in an even layer on a standard cookie sheet so that they do not overlap. Toast pecans for about 10 minutes, or until fragrant and flavorful. Watch carefully so that they do not burn. Once toasted, remove from cookie sheet and set aside until cool. Toss the toasted pecans into a food processor and pulse just until crumbly. Don't overmix.

- In a medium bowl, sift together sorghum flour, potato starch, baking powder, and xanthan gum. Stir in the pulsed pecans.

- In a separate mixing bowl, cream together the margarine and sugar until smooth.

- In a small bowl, combine the flaxseed meal with the water and let rest until gelled, for about 5 minutes. Fold in prepared flaxseed meal with the margarine mixture and mix until combined. Gradually add in the flour mixture, adding up to ⅓ cup additional sorghum flour until the dough can be easily handled. Shape into two separate disks and chill until cold.

- Once the dough is well chilled, take one of the disks and place it in between two pieces of parchment paper and roll until large enough to cover the baking pan.

- Transfer the dough to cover the bottom of the pan, gently pushing down the edges to form a wall around the crust. Spread the blueberry preserves evenly over the layer of crust.

- Take the second disk of dough and crumble into small pieces. Top the jam liberally with dough crumbles. Chill the pan in your freezer while you preheat oven to 350°F.

- Bake for about 35 minutes or until crust becomes golden brown.

- Let cool, then slice into squares. Store bars in an airtight container in refrigerator for up to 1 week.

PEANUT BUTTER MAPLE CRISPY TREATS

YIELD: 12 BARS

I never tire of crispy rice treats. These feature peanut butter and are lightly painted with melted chocolate to give them extra oomph! Try these with chocolate hazelnut butter (Justin's is a great choice) instead of peanut butter. Then just try not to eat the whole pan yourself.

3 tablespoons coconut oil
4 cups vegan marshmallows, such as Dandies
1 teaspoon maple extract
2 tablespoons maple syrup
½ cup smooth peanut butter
6 cups gluten-free crispy rice cereal
1 cup non dairy chocolate chips

- Lightly grease an 8 × 8-inch baking dish using either margarine or coconut oil.

- In a large saucepan over medium heat, melt the 3 tablespoons coconut oil slightly so that the bottom of the saucepan is coated. Add the marshmallows and heat over medium heat until mostly melted, stirring often to prevent burning. Stir in the maple extract, maple syrup, and peanut butter and continue to stir until completely incorporated.

- Place crispy rice cereal into a large bowl and pour hot marshmallow mixture over the crispy rice cereal. Mix quickly to ensure that all the cereal is coated with marshmallow mixture. Spread mixture into the prepared pan and press down firmly using greased hands. Let set until hardened, for about 2 hours. Cut into 2 × 2-inch squares.

- Melt chocolate over double boiler and drizzle the chocolate onto all sides of the bars and place onto waxed paper or a silicone mat. Let chocolate harden completely before enjoying. Store in airtight container for up to 1 week.

TOFFEE CRACKER COOKIES

YIELD: 24 COOKIES

Utilizing crunchy crackers, these cookie bars have a salty and sweet flavor with a candy-like crunch. Out of crackers? You can also use plain cookies to make these; opt for a crunchy cookie such as vanilla wafers or graham crackers.

4 to 5 ounces (about 25 crackers) gluten-free, egg-free crackers, such as Glutino's table crackers
½ cup non dairy margarine
½ cup brown sugar
1 cup semi-sweet non dairy chocolate chips
½ cup sliced toasted almonds or pecans

- Preheat oven to 400°F. Line a medium (about 9 × 13 inches) lipped cookie sheet or baking pan with parchment paper.

- Arrange the crackers on the parchment, as best as you can, in a single layer. Small gaps in between are fine.

- In a 2-quart saucepan, bring together the margarine and brown sugar over medium heat. Stir often, and bring to a boil. Once it hits a boil, let cook for 3 minutes, without stirring. Carefully and strategically pour the hot candy syrup over the crackers to cover. Bake for 5 minutes. Immediately remove from the oven and sprinkle the chocolate chips to cover. Let set for about 4 minutes, and then spread the chocolate to evenly cover the candy. Sprinkle with the almonds. Let rest for 1 hour in a cool place. Freeze briefly until candy has hardened and then cut into squares. Store in airtight container for up to 1 week.

Chapter 4

LUSCIOUS PIES, PASTRIES, TARTS, AND CHEESECAKES

Baking pies is a wonderful hobby because with just a little bit of extra effort, you end up with a dessert that is so impressive it just begs to be shared. I recommend not trying to bake pies that use the Flakey Classic Pie Crust or Puff Pastry on especially humid days, as the tendency for the dough to stick will be much greater, resulting in a frustrating pie baking experience. Shoot for cooler or dry summer days instead for perfect pies every time.

BASICS

FLAKEY CLASSIC PIE CRUST

YIELD: 2 STANDARD-SIZE PIE CRUSTS, OR ENOUGH FOR 1 LATTICE-TOPPED OR COVERED PIE

This piecrust is a staple in this chapter. With a flaky, buttery consistency, it truly does make a pie stand out!

1 cup superfine brown rice flour
¾ cup white rice flour
½ cup potato starch
½ cup tapioca flour
1½ teaspoons xanthan gum
½ teaspoon baking powder
3 tablespoons sugar
10 tablespoons cold non dairy margarine
3 tablespoons lemon juice
½ cup ice-cold water

- In a large bowl, whisk together the superfine brown rice flour, white rice flour, potato starch, tapioca flour, xanthan gum, baking powder, and sugar.

- Drop the margarine into the flour mixture by tablespoons. Use fingers or pastry blender to quickly mix into an even crumble. Using a large fork, stir in the lemon juice and cold water until a soft dough forms. If the dough seems too sticky, add a touch more brown rice flour. Wrap in plastic wrap and chill in the freezer for 15 minutes, or refrigerator for at least 1 hour before using.

- Keeps tightly covered in refrigerator for up to 1 week, and frozen for up to 3 months.

This crust freezes well, so feel free to shape the unbaked dough into a patty and place into two freezer-safe bags (double layered), and, the day before using, allow to thaw in refrigerator overnight before rolling out to use in a recipe. Or roll it out onto two aluminum pie pans, cover in plastic wrap, and freeze. Pie makin' is easy if you already have the crusts prepared ahead of time!

PUFF PASTRY

YIELD: 20 SERVINGS

The key to this super-flakey pastry is keeping the dough cold! Be sure to chill adequately between rotations to ensure a workable dough. I also recommend chilling all ingredients before getting started.

¾ cup superfine brown rice flour
¾ cup white rice flour
⅔ cup potato starch
⅓ cup tapioca flour
2 teaspoons xanthan gum
1¼ cups very cold non dairy margarine
½ cup ice-cold water

- In a large bowl, whisk together the brown rice flour, ½ cup of the white rice flour, potato starch, tapioca flour, and xanthan gum. Drop in the margarine by the spoonful. Using clean hands, quickly cut the margarine into the flour until the mixture resembles pebbles.

- Add in the cold water and mix quickly to form a slightly sticky dough. Punch down into the bowl to flatten the dough and sprinkle with 2 tablespoons white rice flour; pat into the dough to make it less sticky. Flip and repeat with the additional 2 tablespoons white rice flour.

- Chill the dough for 20 minutes in the freezer.

- In between two sheets of parchment paper, roll out the dough into a rectangle about 5 × 9 inches. Use a straight edge to square up the edges, forming a solid rectangle. Work quickly so that the dough stays cold!

- Fold the dough into thirds (like folding a letter) and rotate a quarter of a turn. Use the parchment to help fold the dough over evenly. Roll it out again into another rectangle 5 × 9 inches. Fold it into thirds once again. Wrap loosely in parchment and chill in the freezer for an additional 20 minutes.

- Repeat the steps again, exactly as described above. Wrap and chill the puff pastry until ready to use. When working with the pastry, be sure not to roll it out too thin, ⅓ to ½ of an inch is just right.

154

- Use as directed in recipes calling for puff pastry. To deepen the color of the pastry, mix 2 teaspoons cornstarch with ½ cup water—bring to a boil over medium heat and cook until translucent. Brush a little of the paste onto the surface before baking. Keeps frozen for up to 1 month.

EASY PUFF COOKIES

Preheat oven to 400°F. Dust a sheet of parchment with turbinado sugar. Place the puff pastry dough onto the sugared surface and dust with more sugar. Place another sheet of parchment onto the dough and roll out to ⅓ to ½ inch thick. Use a fun cookie cutter to cut out shapes.

Bake on a parchment-covered cookie sheet for about 20 minutes, until golden brown.

PIES

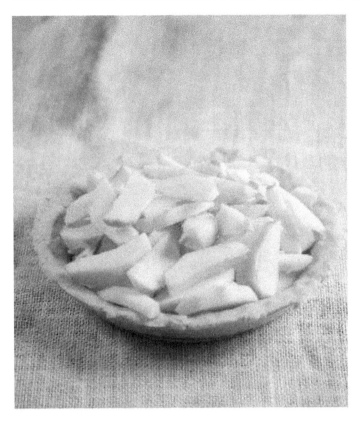

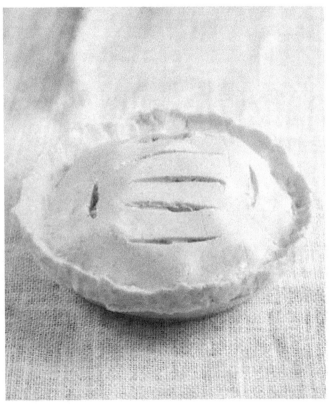

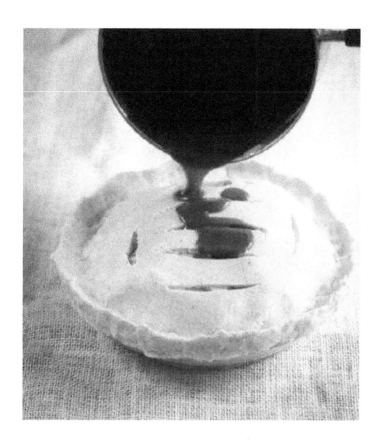

SUGAR CRUNCH APPLE PIE

YIELD: 8 SERVINGS

Adding the sugary syrup to the assembled pie is fun and delicious, as it creates a crisp sugar topping, not unlike the candy crunch from crème brûlée.

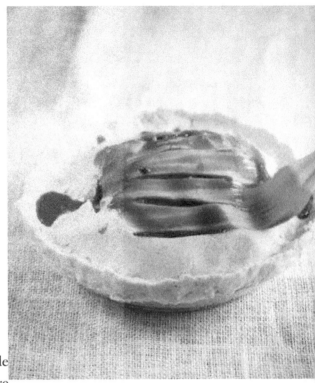

1 recipe Flakey Classic Piecrust

APPLES

8 medium Granny Smith apples

½ teaspoon cardamom

1 teaspoon cinnamon

½ teaspoon cloves

SAUCE

½ cup non dairy margarine

4 tablespoons superfine brown rice flour

¼ cup water

1 cup packed brown sugar

- Prepare the pie dough according to recipe directions, divide into two disks and chill for 2 hours in your refrigerator. Core and peel the apples. Slice thinly and lightly toss with cardamom, cinnamon, and cloves.

- Once pie crusts are chilled, roll out one section of dough in between two sheets of parchment paper to a ¼ inch thickness. Use the parchment paper to help flip the rolled out crust into a lightly greased pie pan. Cut off excess dough and reserve.

- Heap the sliced apples into a mound on top of the crust in the pie pan.

- Take the second chilled dough disk and roll to same thickness in between two sheets of parchment paper. As you did with the first crust, use the parchment to help you flip the dough over on top of the mound of apples. If any dough rips, simply use your fingertips dipped in water to help seal it back together. Build up the sides with excess dough to form a shallow wall as the outer crust. Make a few ¼-inch-wide slits in the top crust to vent.

- Whisk the ingredients for the sauce together into a 2-quart saucepan on medium heat and let it come to a boil, while stirring occasionally. After it has come to a boil, reduce heat to simmer and let cook for 2 minutes. Remove the sauce from the heat.

- Preheat your oven to 425°F. Pour the sugar mixture on top of pie crust, aiming mostly for the slits in the center, and allow any excess to drip over sides. Once all sauce has been added to the pie use a pastry brush to gently brush the remaining syrup evenly over the pie.

- Bake for 15 minutes, then reduce oven temp to 350°F and bake for an additional 35 to 45 minutes. Remove from oven, and let cool for at least 2 hours before serving. Store in airtight container for up to 2 days.

BANANA CREAM PIE

YIELD: 10 SERVINGS

Up until the Great Depression, bananas were practically unheard of in desserts. Apparently, it was the frugalness of using the overripe bananas that led to incorporating them into sweets. With its rich, cream filling, this pie is the very opposite of frugal! It is best enjoyed right after cooling as the bananas tend to discolor after a day or so; one very good way to remedy this is to freeze the pie immediately after it cools and serve mostly frozen.

½ recipe Flakey Classic Pie Crust

FILLING

¾ cup sugar

⅓ cup white rice flour

¼ teaspoon salt

2 cups non dairy milk

3 tablespoons cornstarch mixed with 3 tablespoons water

2 tablespoons non dairy margarine

2 teaspoons vanilla extract

4 large bananas

- Preheat oven to 400°F.

- Prepare the pie crust according to recipe directions and then blind bake in oven for 10 minutes. Reduce oven temperature to 350°F.

- In a 2-quart saucepan, whisk together the sugar, white rice flour, salt, nondairy milk, and cornstarch slurry. Add the margarine and vanilla extract. Heat over medium heat until the mixture comes to a boil, stirring constantly. Let cook for 1 minute, still stirring constantly, until the mixture thickens considerably.

- Slice the bananas into the baked pie crust forming an even layer. Pour the hot sugar mixture over the bananas to cover and bake in preheated oven for 15 minutes. Remove from oven and let cool. Chill and serve with fresh banana slices and Sweetened Whipped Coconut Cream. Store in airtight container in refrigerator for up to 2 days.

KEY LIME PIE

YIELD: 10 SERVINGS

Sweet yet sour, this creamy pie will transport you straight to the Florida Keys. I recommend using bottled key lime juice for ease and availability.

CRUST

1 cup gluten-free cookie crumbs (use hard cookie such as Pizzelles, Cinnamon Graham Crackers, Vanilla Wafers, etc.)

1 cup ground pecans

3 tablespoons sugar

2 tablespoons ground chia seed mixed with 4 tablespoons water

1 tablespoon coconut oil

FILLING

1 (350 g) package extra-firm silken tofu

1 cup key lime juice

1 cup canned full-fat coconut milk

½ cup coconut cream from the top of a can of full-fat coconut milk

1 cup sugar

2 tablespoons confectioners sugar

¾ teaspoons salt

¼ cup besan/chickpea flour

¼ cup white rice flour

2 tablespoons cornstarch

1 teaspoon lime zest, plus more for topping

- Preheat oven to 375°F.

- Mix together all the crust ingredients, in order given, and press into a standard-size pie pan.

- In the bowl of a food processor, place the filling ingredients, pulsing a few times after each addition, until smooth. Be sure to scrape down sides as needed.

- Pour the filling mixture into the crust and carefully transfer to the middle rack of your oven. Bake for 20 minutes. Reduce heat to 300°F and bake for an additional 40 to 45 minutes, until very lightly golden brown on edges. Let cool at room temperature and then chill in refrigerator overnight. Top with lime zest and Sweetened Whipped Coconut Cream. Store in airtight container in refrigerator for up to 2 days.

ALLERGY NOTE

If you have a nut allergy and would like to make this pie, simply swap out the pecans in the crust for toasted sunflower or pumpkin seeds.

PUMPKIN PIE

YIELD: 10 SERVINGS

Popular during the autumn months, pumpkin pie didn't become the traditional dessert of Thanksgiving until the early 1800s. This pumpkin pie is just like the ones my mother used to make for the holiday—with a crust that's softer on the bottom and crispy on the sides. Strange as it sounds, that was always my favorite part of the pie!

½ recipe Flakey Classic Pie Crust

1 cup sugar

1 teaspoon cinnamon

1 teaspoon ginger

½ teaspoon ground cloves

¼ teaspoon ground nutmeg

1 teaspoon salt

1 (350 g) package extra-firm silken tofu

1½ teaspoons vanilla extract

⅓ cup superfine brown rice flour

2 cups canned pumpkin puree

¼ cup apple cider or nondairy milk

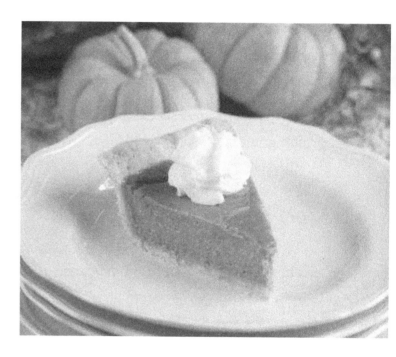

- Prepare the pie crust according to recipe directions. Shape the dough into a disk and chill in the refrigerator for at least 1 hour.

- Preheat oven to 425°F. Roll out the crust in between two pieces of parchment and then flip over to lay the pie crust evenly into the bottom of a standard-size pie pan. Pinch the top to make the pie fancy, or flute.

- Combine all the ingredients for the pie filling in a food processor and blend until very smooth. Spread pie filling into unbaked crust and bake for 15 minutes.

- Reduce your oven temperature to 350°F and bake for an additional 40 minutes, or until the crust is golden brown. Let pie cool completely and refrigerate for at least 4 hours before serving. This pie is best when chilled overnight. Store in airtight container in refrigerator for up to 5 days.

STRAWBERRY PIE

YIELD: 10 SERVINGS

Strawberry Pie always reminds me of the beginning of summertime, right when the weather gets warm enough to start craving cold desserts. This is a great recipe to make the night before as it needs to firm up for quite some time, plus it is excellent served very cold.

½ recipe Flakey Classic Piecrust

FILLING

4 cups strawberries, sliced

1 cup granulated sugar

4 tablespoons cornstarch

¼ cup water Pinch salt

2 or 3 sliced strawberries for a garnish

- Preheat oven to 425°F. Lightly grease a standard-size pie pan and dust with brown rice or sorghum flour.

- Prepare the pie crust according to recipe directions.

- Roll out the dough in between two pieces of parchment paper until it is about ¼ inch thick. Carefully invert onto a pie pan, shaping to fit and make a lip on the crust. Using a fork, poke about twenty small holes evenly over the crust. Bake for 20 minutes, or until crust is firm. Let cool completely before filling.

- Filling: Place 1½ cups of the strawberries plus the sugar into a 2-quart saucepan and mash gently with a potato masher. Cook over medium heat just until sugar dissolves completely.

- In a medium bowl, whisk together the cornstarch and water until smooth and add to the cooked strawberry mixture along with the salt. Bring to a boil over medium heat and allow to cook for about 2 minutes. Remove from heat and let cool slightly, but not completely, for about 15 minutes. Arrange the remaining 2½ cups strawberries evenly into the piecrust. Pour the cooked filling into prepared pie pan and let chill in fridge until firm, for about 12 hours. Garnish with additional strawberry slices. Serve cold. Store in airtight container in refrigerator for up to 2 days.

CHERRY PIE

YIELD: 10 SERVINGS

I recommend using Bing or sour cherries for this pie to achieve that lovely deep red color that we're so accustomed to with cherry pie. I particularly love this pie served warm from the oven à la mode.

1 recipe Flakey Classic Piecrust
4 cups fresh cherries, pitted
¼ cup tapioca flour 1 cup sugar
¼ teaspoon salt
1 teaspoon vanilla extract
4 teaspoons non dairy margarine

- Prepare the pie crust according to recipe directions and divide crust evenly into two sections. Refrigerate one disk while you roll out the other in between two sheets of parchment paper, to about ¼ inch thickness. Flip over into a deep-dish pie pan and shape to fit the pan.

- In a large bowl, toss the cherries with the tapioca flour, sugar, salt, and vanilla extract until evenly coated. Place into the pie shell and spread evenly. Dot with margarine. Roll out the other half of the crust in between two sheets of parchment paper to ¼ inch thickness. Drape over the top of the pie, inverting using one sheet of parchment to assist, and top the pie with the second crust. Flute the edges to seal and then slice a few small slits in the crust to vent. Bake for 45 to 50 minutes, until pie crust is golden brown. Let pie cool slightly before serving. Store in airtight container for up to 2 days.

You can use frozen cherries if fresh aren't in season; simply thaw them out and drain thoroughly before using.

ANY BERRY PIE

YIELD: 10 SERVINGS

Blackberry, blueberry, raspberry … any type of berry can be used in this pie and it will still be delicious. My favorite is a solid tie between blackberry and blueberry.

1 recipe Flakey Classic Piecrust
½ cup brown sugar
¼ cup sugar
3 tablespoons cornstarch
½ teaspoon salt
1 teaspoon vanilla extract
4 cups blackberries, blueberries, or raspberries
1 tablespoon non dairy margarine

- Preheat oven to 425°F.

- Prepare the crust according to recipe directions and roll out half of the crust in between two sheets of parchment to ¼ inch thick, while keeping the other half chilled. Place one half of crust into a deep-dish pie pan and shape to fit the pie pan.

- In a medium bowl, toss together the brown sugar, sugar, cornstarch, and salt until well mixed. Add in the vanilla extract and berries and gently stir until the berries are completed covered. Place berries into the piecrust and dot evenly with margarine.

- Roll out the other half of pie crust in between two sheets of parchment until about ¼ inch thick. Work fast! Have a pizza cutter handy and slice 1 × 9- inch strips of pie crust. Use your hands to gently peel up the tip of the strip and drape on top of the blueberries to form a crosshatch pattern until pie is covered to your liking. You can also use a cookie cutter to cut out shapes to top the pie.

- Bake for 40 minutes, or until the piecrust is deep golden brown, but not burned. Serve hot à la mode or room temperature. Store in airtight container for up to 2 days.

TARTE TATIN

YIELD: 8 SERVINGS

This recipe is super simple but requires a pan that can safely, and effectively, go from stove top to oven, such as cast iron. For a perfect Tarte Tatin, choose a variety of apple that will hold its shape while cooking, such as Granny Smith or Gala.

½ recipe Flakey Classic Piecrust
¼ cup non dairy margarine
½ cup brown sugar
5 small apples, peeled, cored, and quartered

- Preheat oven to 425°F. Shape the pie crust dough into a disk and chill until ready to use.

- Over medium heat, in a 9-inch cast-iron pan, melt the margarine until liquid. Sprinkle on the brown sugar and then place the apples directly on top of the sugar, arranging snugly and evenly so that the domed sides are facing down. Try to eliminate any excess spaces in between the apples. Let the apples cook, completely undisturbed over medium heat for 20 minutes.

- Transfer the hot pan to the oven and bake on the middle rack for 20 more minutes.

- Remove from oven and let rest briefly.

- Roll the pie crust out in between two sheets of parchment paper, just wide enough to cover the cast-iron pan with about 1 inch excess. Flip the piecrust over the apples to cover, and push the dough gently down to form a rustic top crust. Bake for an additional 20 minutes, and then remove from oven and let cool for 10 minutes.

- Flip the pie out onto a lipped plate, roughly the same size as the tart. The dough will invert to form a lovely crust. If any apples happen to stick to the pan, carefully remove and place them back onto the tart.

- Serve warm or room temperature. Store in airtight container for up to 2 days.

CHOCOLATE SILK PIE

YIELD: 10 SERVINGS

This is one of my favorite desserts to bring to potlucks because of its simplicity and versatility. The secret ingredient is silken tofu, which creates a base that's both firm and silky. Top each individual piece with Sweetened Whipped Coconut Cream just before serving.

½ recipe Flakey Classic Piecrust

2 (350 g) packages extra-firm silken tofu

2 teaspoons vanilla extract

2 tablespoons cocoa powder (I like extra-dark)

½ cup sugar

1½ cups chopped non dairy chocolate or chocolate chips

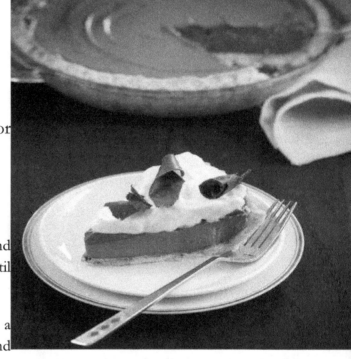

- Preheat oven to 400°F.

- Prepare the pie crust according to recipe directions and roll out in between two sheets of parchment paper until about ¼ inch thick.

- Flip over the parchment to gently place the crust into a standard-size glass pie pan. Fold or flute the crust and pierce bottom several times evenly with fork. Bake for 20 minutes, or until light golden brown. Remove from oven.

- To prepare the filling, blend the tofu, vanilla extract, cocoa powder, and sugar in a food processor until completely smooth, scraping down sides as needed.

- In a double boiler, melt the chocolate and drizzle into the tofu mixture and blend until completely incorporated. Spread filling into baked pie shell and let cool at room temperature for 1 hour before transferring to the refrigerator to chill until slightly firm, 4 hours up to overnight. Store in airtight container in refrigerator for up to 3 days.

SKY-HIGH PEANUT BUTTER PIE

YIELD: 10 SERVINGS

If you love peanut butter you're going to flip over this pie. Rich peanut butter and chocolate combine for a luscious base, while fluffy coconut cream gives the pie its name. You can also switch this up and use almond or cashew butter if you have a peanut allergy.

½ recipe Flakey Classic Piecrust

4 ounces semi-sweet chocolate

3 (350 g) packages firm silken tofu

2 cups creamy peanut butter

2 cups confectioners sugar

3 tablespoons ground chia seed

½ teaspoon sea salt

1 recipe Sweetened Whipped Coconut Cream

2 ounces non dairy chocolate chips or chunks, melted, for drizzling

¼ cup crushed roasted and salted peanuts

- Preheat oven to 400°F and prepare the pie crust according to recipe directions. Roll out in between two sheets of parchment until ¼ inch thick. Drape over a deep-dish pie pan and press down evenly to cover. Flute edges and bake for 20 minutes, or until lightly golden brown. Remove from oven and place on wire rack to cool. Sprinkle 4 ounces of the chocolate chips evenly onto the piecrust and let rest for 5 minutes. Spread the melted chocolate, using a silicone spatula, to coat the inside of the pie crust. Let cool completely until chocolate is rehardened—once the crust is at room temperature, place in the refrigerator to speed up the process.

- In a food processor combine the tofu, peanut butter, sugar, chia seed, and salt. Blend until completely smooth, for about 5 minutes. Spread into the prepared pie crust, and freeze for at least 3 hours. Transfer to refrigerator and chill overnight. Before serving, top with whipped coconut cream and drizzle with chocolate. Sprinkle with crushed peanuts. Store in an airtight container in the refrigerator for up to 2 days.

PECAN PIE

YIELD: 10 SERVINGS

The first time I tasted Pecan Pie, I was smitten. Even today when I get around one, it takes a bit of restraint for me to stop eating the whole darn thing! Best to share with others, or just make two pies, and save yourself the heartache.

½ recipe Flakey Classic Piecrust
2 tablespoons flaxseed meal
¼ cup water
1¼ cups packed brown sugar
2 tablespoons superfine brown rice flour, or white rice flour
2 teaspoons vanilla extract
½ cup melted non dairy margarine
1½ cups chopped pecans

- Preheat oven to 400°F. Prepare the pie crust according to recipe directions and press into a standard-size pie pan, making the crust slightly shorter than the top edge of the pan. Flute or use a spoon to make a design in the top of the crust.

- In a large bowl, stir together flaxseed meal and water and let set for 5 minutes, until gelled. Transfer to a mixing bowl and whip on high speed using a whisk attachment for 1 minute (or using elbow grease and a whisk), until fluffy. Add the sugar, brown rice flour, vanilla extract, and margarine. Fold in 1 cup of the chopped pecans. Stir well. Spoon filling into unbaked crust and then top with remaining chopped pecans.

- Bake for 35 to 40 minutes, until crust is golden brown and filling is bubbly. Carefully remove from the oven and let cool completely, for at least 4 hours, before serving. Store in airtight container in refrigerator for up to 2 days.

CHEESECAKES

NEW YORK–STYLE CHEESECAKE

YIELD: 12 SERVINGS

This cheesecake takes a little added patience as it absolutely must be left in the oven 1 to 2 hours to finish baking and then it must be chilled overnight, but it is so worth it. This classic dessert is just perfect plain but pairs exceptionally well with fruit topping. Try it with Cherry Vanilla Compote, Broiled Persimmons, Blueberry Lavender Jam, or even plain fruit such as strawberries.

¼ cup almond meal

4 (8-ounce) tubs nondairy cream cheese, such as Tofutti brand

1¾ cups sugar

½ cup non dairy sour cream or coconut cream

½ cup besan/chickpea flour mixed with ½ cup water

¼ cup superfine brown rice flour or white rice flour

1 teaspoon vanilla extract

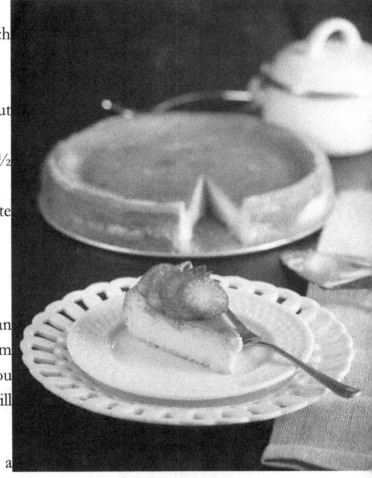

- Preheat oven to 350°F and lightly grease an 8-inch springform pan. Sprinkle the bottom of the pan evenly with the almond meal. You may use a larger pan, but your cheesecake will be thinner and may need to cook less time.

- Place all the remaining ingredients into a food processor and blend until very smooth, for about 2 minutes, scraping down the sides as needed. Don't taste the batter as the besan will make it unpleasant until baked!

- Bake for 45 minutes at 350°F and then reduce heat to 325°F. Bake for an additional 35 minutes, and then turn off oven. Let the cheesecake cool, inside the closed oven, for about 1 to 2 hours. Chill overnight before serving. Store in airtight container in refrigerator for up to 4 days.

PISTACHIO ROSE CHEESECAKE

YIELD: 10 SERVINGS

This fragrant cake is delightful when served with a dollop of Sweetened Whipped Coconut Cream and a dry white wine, or sparkling grape juice for the kids. Rose water can be located in most specialty grocers near other similar extracts and flavorings. Certainly, if you cannot locate this particular flavoring, equal amounts of spiced rum or vanilla extract would replace it just fine, albeit without the floral undertones.

CRUST

1 tablespoon flaxseed meal

2 tablespoons water

1 cup pistachios, pulsed until crumbly

2 tablespoons sugar

1 tablespoon almond or canola oil

¼ cup almond meal, plus extra for sprinkling

FILLING

2 cups (20 ounces) silken tofu

1 to 1½ teaspoons rose water (the more the rosier!)

3 (8-ounce) containers nondairy cream cheese, such as Tofutti

¾ cup sugar

¼ teaspoon salt

3 tablespoons white rice flour

2 drops pink food coloring (optional)

- Preheat oven to 400°F. Lightly grease only the sides of an 8-inch springform pan. You may use a larger pan, but your cheesecake will be thinner and may need to cook less time.

- In a small bowl, combine flaxseed meal with water and let rest until gelled, for about 5 minutes. In a large bowl, mix together the pistachios, sugar, almond oil, almond meal, and prepared flaxseed meal until clumpy. Use very lightly greased hands and press firmly into the bottom of the springform pan and cover as best as you can. Once it is spread out covering as much surface as possible, sprinkle lightly with almond meal and then press down to cover completely and evenly.

- In a food processor, combine all the ingredients for the filling and blend until completely smooth, for about 5 minutes, scraping down sides often. Spread the filling evenly into the prepared springform pan and then bake for 15 minutes.

- Reduce heat to 250°F, without removing the cheesecake from the oven, and bake for an additional 60 minutes. Turn oven off and let cheesecake remain for 1 more hour. Let cool for 1 hour at room temperature on a wire rack and then transfer to the refrigerator to cool overnight. Store in airtight container in refrigerator for up to 4 days.

CARAMEL CHAI CHEESECAKE

YIELD: 10 SERVINGS

This version of the classic dessert is pure decadence. If you really love cinnamon, cloves, and allspice, serve it with a piping-hot mug of chai for the ultimate spicy indulgence.

CRUST

6 ounces (170 g) pecans
3 tablespoons melted non dairy margarine
3 tablespoons sugar
2 tablespoons superfine brown rice flour

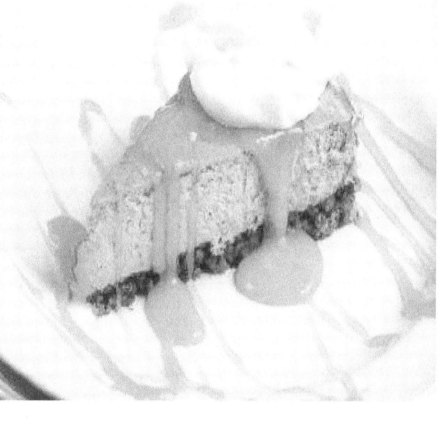

FILLING

1 (350 g) package extra-firm silken tofu
3 (8-ounce) tubs nondairy cream cheese, such as Tofutti
⅔ cup packed light brown sugar
5 tablespoons superfine brown rice flour
¼ teaspoon sea salt
1 teaspoon cinnamon
⅛ teaspoon allspice
¼ teaspoon ground black pepper
¼ teaspoon ground cloves
⅛ teaspoon cardamom
1 teaspoon vanilla extract
1 recipe Caramel Sauce

For the Crust

- Preheat oven to 400°F. Pulse the pecans in a food processor, just until crumbly. Stir in the rest of the crust ingredients and press (using hands dusted with superfine brown rice flour) into an 8-inch springform pan.

- Bake for 10 minutes and then remove from the oven.

For the Filling

- Place all the ingredients for the filling into a food processor and blend until very smooth, for at least 5 minutes. Spread onto the prepared crust and bake in preheated oven for 15 minutes.

- Reduce heat to 250°F and allow cheesecake to bake for an additional 60 minutes. Turn oven off and let cool for up to 2 more hours while remaining in the oven. Chill in refrigerator overnight and then make the Caramel Sauce just before serving, so that you have hot caramel sauce on a cold cheesecake. Top with Sweetened Whipped Coconut Cream. Store in airtight container in refrigerator for up to 4 days.

PUMPKIN PECAN CHEESECAKE

YIELD: 12 SERVINGS

What could be more apropos for autumn than this flavor combo? If you're looking for a wonderful alternative (or addition!) to Pumpkin Pie on Thanksgiving, look no further.

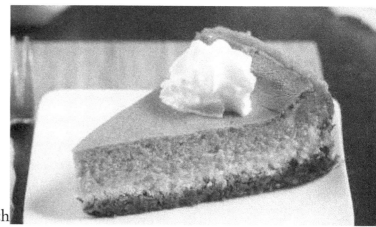

CRUST
1 tablespoon flaxseed meal
2 tablespoons water
2 cups pecans
¼ teaspoon salt
¼ cup brown sugar
FILLING
1 block firm silken tofu
2 (8-ounce) tubs nondairy cream cheese, such as Tofutti
1 cup sugar
¼ cup plus 2 tablespoons brown rice flour
¼ cup lemon juice
1 (15-ounce) can pumpkin puree
⅓ cup brown sugar
1 teaspoon cinnamon
½ teaspoon pumpkin pie spice

- Preheat oven to 400°F. Lightly grease the sides of an 8-inch springform pan.

- In a small bowl, mix together the flaxseed meal and the water. Let rest for 5 minutes, until gelled. In a food processor, pulse together the pecans, salt, and brown sugar until the mixture resembles coarse crumbles. Add in prepared flaxseed meal and pulse again until pecans come together into a loose dough. Press into the bottom of the prepared springform pan and bake for 10 minutes.

- In the meantime, clean the food processor and mix together the tofu, non dairy cream cheese, sugar, ¼ cup brown rice flour, and lemon juice. Blend until completely smooth, for about 2 minutes, scraping down sides as needed. Scoop out about 1 cup of this mixture and spread evenly onto the crust to form a thin white layer.

- Add the canned pumpkin, brown sugar, cinnamon, pumpkin pie spice, and remaining 2 tablespoons brown rice flour. Blend again until completely smooth, scraping down sides as needed. Spread on top of white layer.

- Bake for 15 minutes. Reduce oven temperature to 325°F and bake for an additional hour. Turn oven off and let cheesecake remain for about 1 hour. Chill completely overnight before serving. Store in airtight container in refrigerator for up to 3 days.

CHOCOLATE BROWNIE CHEESECAKE

YIELD: 10 SERVINGS

This cheesecake has a super-secret special ingredient: black beans! But you can't tell—in gluten-free baking, oftentimes beans and legumes can be our best friends, providing a little bit of rise and a lot of binding power, along with a totally neutral flavor, so you won't taste anything but chocolaty goodness.

CRUST

1 cup hazelnut meal (finely ground hazelnuts)

2 tablespoons cocoa powder

3 tablespoons sugar

3 tablespoons melted non dairy margarine or coconut oil

FILLING

⅔ cup sugar

3 (8-ounce) tubs nondairy cream cheese, such as Tofutti

1 cup canned black beans, drained and rinsed

½ cup non dairy milk

¼ cup brown rice flour

2 cups non dairy chocolate chips, melted

- Grease the sides of an 8-inch springform pan and preheat oven to 400°F.

- In a small bowl, stir together the hazelnut meal, cocoa powder, and sugar. Drizzle in the melted margarine and stir to combine. Press the mixture onto the bottom of the springform pan to form an even layer. Bake for 9 minutes. Remove from oven and decrease temperature to 375°F.

- In a food processor, combine all the ingredients for the filling, one at a time, in the order listed, making sure that all the ingredients have been completely blended before adding in the melted chocolate chips.

- Spread filling mixture evenly on top of the prebaked crust. Bake for 30 minutes, and then reduce oven temperature to 325°F. Bake for an additional 40 minutes. Turn oven off and allow cheesecake to remain for 2 hours. Chill completely—overnight is best—before serving. Store in airtight container in refrigerator for up to 4 days.

TARTS, COBBLERS, AND PASTRIES

CHOCOLATE PISTACHIO TART

YIELD: 8 SERVINGS

I love the contrast of the deep chocolate filling against
the salty pistachio crust. This pie freezes beautifully and
can be thawed in the refrigerator overnight the day before
serving.

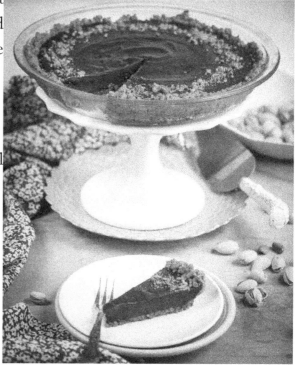

CRUST

2 tablespoons flaxseed meal 3 tablespoons water

1 cup pistachios, pulsed until crumbly (plus additional
crushed pistachios for garnish)

3 tablespoons fine yellow cornmeal

2 scant tablespoons sugar

½ teaspoon salt

3 tablespoons olive oil

FILLING

2½ cups nondairy semi-sweet chocolate chips

1⅓ cups coconut milk

1 teaspoon vanilla extract

⅛ teaspoon ground cumin

¼ teaspoon sea salt

- Preheat oven to 400°F.

- In a small bowl, combine the flaxseed meal with the water and let rest until gelled, for
  about 5 minutes. In a separate small bowl, whisk together the pistachios, cornmeal, sugar,
  and salt until well combined. Evenly mix in the olive oil and flaxseed gel, using clean
  hands.

- Press crust into a standard-size pie pan, about ⅛ inch thick. Bake for 10 minutes.
  Remove and let cool completely.

- To make the filling, place the chocolate chips in a large heat-safe bowl.

- In a small saucepan, combine the coconut milk, vanilla extract, cumin, and salt and bring
  just to a boil over medium heat. Once bubbly, pour over chocolate chips and mix well.
  Spread the chocolate mixture into the piecrust and let cool at room temperature, for
  about 1 hour. Sprinkle with crushed pistachios and transfer into the refrigerator to cool
  completely until firm. Store in airtight container in refrigerator for up to 2 days.

181

PEARBERRY TART

YIELD: 8 SERVINGS

This fruity concoction is pretty and delish! I recommend red raspberries as they look so beautiful against the amber-colored pears. The tart is easy to prep, and it has a silky custard texture that will make you yearn for a second slice!

½ recipe Flakey Classic Piecrust

⅓ cup besan/chickpea flour

3 tablespoons cornstarch

⅓ cup sugar

½ teaspoon salt

1 cup red raspberries or other berry

2 medium pears, peeled, cored, and sliced

⅓ cup turbinado sugar

- Preheat oven to 400°F.

- Prepare the piecrust as directed and chill in refrigerator for 30 minutes. Roll out in between two sheets of parchment paper to about ¼ inch thick. Flip over onto an 8-inch tart shell and press dough into the pan, trimming any excess.

- In a medium bowl, whisk together the besan, cornstarch, sugar, and salt. Rinse the berries and dredge them in the flour mixture to evenly coat. Remove and set aside. Toss the sliced pears into the mixture as well and then rustically (no fancy pattern needed) arrange the pears and berries into the tart shell. Top with an even layer of turbinado sugar. Bake for 35 to 40 minutes, or until crust is golden brown on edges. Store in airtight container in refrigerator for up to 2 days.

ALMOND APPLE TART

YIELD: 4 SERVINGS

This elegant dessert, which features the fragrant combination of almonds and apples, comes together effortlessly if you already have some puff pastry frozen. You'll have a fancy dessert ready to impress in no time flat. This tart also keeps well if refrigerated for up to 1 week; simply reheat at 350°F for 10 minutes and sprinkle with a touch of turbinado sugar before serving.

½ recipe Puff Pastry
2 tablespoons turbinado sugar
1 large Granny Smith apple, peeled and thinly sliced
1 teaspoon lemon or lime juice
½ cup brown sugar, plus 2 tablespoons for sprinkling on top
1 teaspoon vanilla extract
⅛ teaspoon salt
3 tablespoons cornstarch
2 tablespoons almond meal

- Place a rectangle of chilled puff pastry dough in between two sheets of parchment paper and gently roll out into a rectangle about 5 × 8 inches. Transfer the dough to a baking sheet lined with parchment paper or a silicone mat. Crimp up the edges of the crust to form a lip, gently folding the top back onto itself. Sprinkle evenly with the 2 tablespoons turbinado sugar.

- In a medium bowl, toss the apples with the lemon juice, and then with the remaining ingredients, until the apples are well coated. Arrange the apples onto the tart shell in an even layer, overlapping each slice to form a pattern. Sprinkle with the 2 tablespoons brown sugar.

- Bake for 35 to 40 minutes, or until apples are tender and crust is golden brown. Store in airtight container for up to 2 days.

CRANBERRY WHITE CHOCOLATE CITRUS TART

YIELD: 10 SERVINGS

White chocolate and cranberry is a popular combination; the addition of orange here creates a nice tang. You can make your own dairy-free white chocolate for this tart or seek out your favorite brand elsewhere.

CRUST

1¾ cups almond meal

¼ cup brown sugar

3 tablespoons coconut oil, liquid

Dash salt

TOPPING

1½ cups fresh cranberries

¼ cup sugar

FILLING

2 cups raw cashews, soaked at least 3 hours and drained

¼ cup sugar

½ cup orange juice

1 teaspoon orange zest

5.5 ounces (150 g) non dairy white chocolate

For the Crust

• Preheat oven to 400°F.

• In a small bowl, mix together the almond meal and brown sugar. Stir in the melted coconut oil and salt until completely mixed. Use lightly greased hands or the bottom of a drinking glass and press the mixture into an 8-inch tart pan.

• Bake the crust for 10 minutes in your preheated oven. Remove from the oven and let cool completely.

For the Topping

• Combine the cranberries and sugar in a small saucepan and cook over medium heat, stirring often, until sugar granules have dissolved completely. Increase temperature slightly to reduce until thickened, for about 5 minutes.

184

For the Filling

- In a food processor, blend the cashews with the sugar, orange juice, and zest until very, very smooth, for about 5 minutes. Over a double boiler, melt the white chocolate and then blend with the rest of the ingredients.

- Quickly spread the cashew filling into the cooled tart crust and top with the cranberry mixture. Gently run a knife through the top of the filling to swirl through. Chill in the refrigerator until firm. Store in airtight container in refrigerator for up to 2 days.

WHITE CHOCOLATE PEANUT BUTTER PRETZEL TARTLETS

YIELD: 12 TARTS

Salty pretzels pair so wonderfully with the combined sweetness of white chocolate and peanut butter and are presented in a cute little tartlet package.

1½ cups crushed gluten-free pretzels
6 tablespoons softened non dairy margarine
2 tablespoons sugar
1 cup non dairy white chocolate chips
½ cup smooth peanut butter
¼ cup canned coconut milk
1 cup non dairy milk

- Preheat oven to 350°F. Gather about twelve 2-inch tart pans and lightly spray with nonstick cooking oil.

- Combine the crushed pretzels, margarine, and sugar together until very well mixed. Make sure there are no lumps of margarine. When pressed, the mixture should hold its shape. You may need to add a touch more margarine if it feels too crumbly … but just about a tablespoon or so.

- Gently press the crumbs into the tart pans, making an even crust that is about ¼ inch thick. Handle with care.

- Bake for about 12 minutes, or until dark golden brown. Remove tart shells from oven and let cool on wire racks.

- Once the crusts are cool, begin making your filling.

- Place white chocolate chips into a medium bowl. In a small saucepan, combine the peanut butter, coconut milk, and nondairy milk and cook over medium heat, stirring constantly using a wire whisk.

- Once the mixture just begins to bubble and is very hot, pour over white chocolate chips, stirring quickly to melt. Spoon into the prepared tart shells, allowing to cool at room temperature for about an hour before transferring to the refrigerator to chill completely. Store in airtight container in refrigerator for up to 2 days.

PEACHY KEEN COBBLER

YIELD: 8 SERVINGS

This cobbler is a perfect way to use up a bunch of fruit, especially when you have a lotta hard peaches rolling around—which tends to happen to me quite often during the summertime (I over purchase and don't want to wait for all of them to ripen!). Any stone fruit can be used; try this recipe with plums or apricots, too!

4 peaches (about 4½ cups) peeled and sliced
½ cup sugar
¼ teaspoon ground allspice
3 tablespoons cornstarch
⅓ cup potato starch
⅓ cup white rice flour
⅓ cup besan/chickpea flour
1 teaspoon xanthan gum
1 teaspoon baking powder
3 tablespoons sugar
6 tablespoons non dairy margarine
¼ cup + 2 tablespoons non dairy milk
1 teaspoon lemon juice

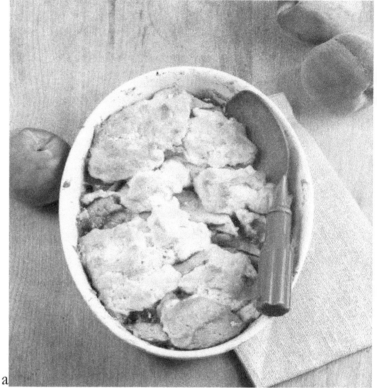

- Preheat oven to 375°F and lightly grease a small stoneware or ceramic baking dish, about 5 × 9 inches.

- In a medium bowl, toss together the peaches, sugar, allspice, and cornstarch. Arrange in the greased baking dish in an even layer.

- In a separate bowl, whisk together the potato starch, white rice flour, besan, xanthan gum, baking powder, and sugar. Cut in the margarine and blend using a pastry blender until even crumbles form. Add in the nondairy milk and lemon juice and stir until smooth.

- Drop by heaping spoonfuls on top of the sliced peaches. Bake for 35 to 40 minutes, or until bubbly and the biscuit top is golden brown on edges. Store in airtight container for up to 1 day.

CHERRY CLAFOUTIS

YIELD: 8 SERVINGS

This recipe is such a perfect use for fresh cherries as this dessert truly accentuates the color and flavor of the short-seasoned fresh fruit. Cherries not in season? Good news: frozen cherries work, too! Thanks to Lydia, who tested for this cookbook, for the tip.

½ block extra-firm tofu, drained but not pressed (about 215 g)
1½ cups besan/chickpea flour
1½ cups non dairy milk
1 teaspoon baking powder
2 tablespoons tapioca flour
¾ cup sugar
¾ teaspoon sea salt
1 teaspoon vanilla extract
2 cups pitted cherries
¼ cup confectioners sugar

- Preheat oven to 350°F and grease an 8-inch cast-iron skillet or glass pie pan with enough margarine to coat.

- Place all the ingredients but the cherries and the confectioner's sugar into a blender and blend until the mixture is uniform and very smooth, scraping down sides as needed. Pour the batter into the prepared pan and then dot evenly with pitted cherries, placing them about ½ inch apart on top of the batter.

- Bake for 50 to 55 minutes, or until a knife inserted into the middle comes out clean. Let cool completely and dust with confectioners sugar before serving. Store in airtight container for up to 2 days in refrigerator.

APPLE CRISP

YIELD: 6 SERVINGS

This simple and rustic dessert is as easy to whip up as it is delicious. Serve à la mode for an over-the-top treat. My favorite type of apple to use in this is Granny Smith, but any crisp variety will do.

5 apples, peeled and sliced ½ to ¼ inch thick
¾ cup brown sugar
½ cup brown rice flour
¼ cup potato starch
1 teaspoon cinnamon
¾ cup certified gluten-free oats
⅓ cup non dairy margarine

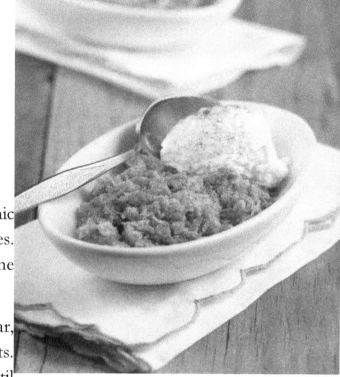

- Preheat oven to 375°F. Lightly grease a ceramic baking dish or cake pan, about 8 × 8 inches. Arrange the sliced apples evenly to cover the bottom of the baking dish.

- In a medium bowl, whisk together the brown sugar, brown rice flour, potato starch, cinnamon, and oats. Cut in the margarine using a pastry blender until crumbly. Sprinkle liberally over the apples.

- Bake for 35 to 40 minutes, until golden brown and bubbly. Store in airtight container in refrigerator for up to 2 days.

MILLE-FEUILLE

YIELD: 8 SERVINGS

Elegant and classy, this French dessert will make your dinner guests do a double take. Even though it looks complicated, it's really quite easy once you have the puff pastry prepared. Just assemble and serve!

½ recipe Puff Pastry
½ recipe Mascarpone
1 cup confectioners sugar
½ cup Strawberry Preserves
¼ cup cacao nibs
½ cup melted chocolate
Strawberries for garnish

- Preheat oven to 400°F. Line a large baking sheet with parchment or a silicone mat. Roll out the puff pastry into a rectangle about ¼ inch thick. Chill briefly in the freezer, for about 10 minutes, and then carefully cut into even-size rectangles, about 2.5 × 4 inches. Using a flat metal spatula, carefully transfer the puff pastry to the prepared baking sheet, about ½ inch apart. Bake for 15 to 20 minutes, until puffed and golden brown. Let cool completely and then assemble the dessert.

- Mix the Mascarpone with the confectioner's sugar and place into a pastry bag equipped with a star tip. Glaze the tops of each pastry rectangles with Strawberry Preserves and then pipe on circles of the Mascarpone mixture until the top of the rectangle is covered. Sprinkle with cacao nibs. Top with another strawberry preserve–glazed pastry rectangle and again, pipe another layer of mascarpone and sprinkle with cacao nibs. Top with a final rectangle of pastry glazed with strawberry preserves and then drizzle with melted chocolate. Top with a halved strawberry. Chill for 1 hour in refrigerator and then serve cold.

MINI MAPLE DONUTS

YIELD: 24 DONUTS

If anything can take me back to the donut shop as a kid, it's these guys. These basic cake donuts have a hint of maple—not too cloying. The glaze also goes well with a variety of other desserts, such as the Devil's Food Cake, Maple Cookies, or even the Classic Chocolate Chip Cookies.

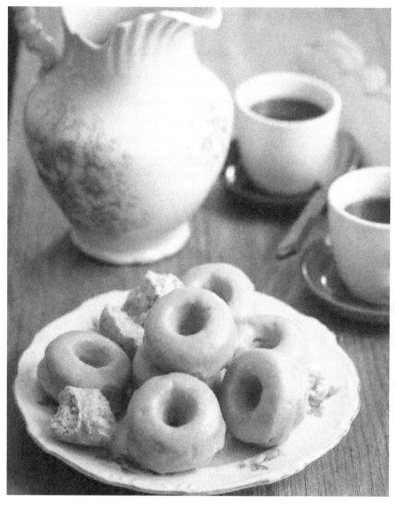

DONUTS

⅓ cup + 2 tablespoons sorghum flour

⅓ cup + 2 tablespoons potato starch

¼ cup tapioca flour

¼ cup brown rice flour

¾ teaspoon xanthan gum

½ teaspoon salt

1 teaspoon baking powder

3 tablespoons olive oil

⅓ cup + 1 tablespoon maple syrup

½ cup brown sugar

⅓ cup + 2 tablespoons non dairy milk

1 tablespoon apple cider vinegar

GLAZE

1¼ cups confectioner's sugar

2 tablespoons non dairy milk

1 teaspoon light corn syrup

1 teaspoon maple syrup

1 teaspoon maple extract

Dash salt

- Preheat oven to 325°F and place your oven rack in the middle of the oven. Lightly grease a mini-size donut pan.

- Combine all the ingredients through the salt into a medium mixing bowl and whisk until well combined. Gradually add in the rest of the donut ingredients, in the order given, and mix well until no lumps remain. You should end up with a tacky batter.

- Fill the cups of the donut pan with batter. Bake for 25 minutes. Let cool completely and then glaze.

- To make the glaze, simply whisk together all ingredients until smooth. Cover cooled donuts completely with glaze and then place onto a wire rack to firm up. Let glaze harden completely before serving. Store in airtight container for up to 4 days.

I like to use corn syrup in my glazes as it truly re-creates that donut-shop texture; however, you may replace the corn syrup with 1 teaspoon maple syrup, which will cause the glaze texture to have a slight variation.

BELGIAN WAFFLES

YIELD: 7 WAFFLES

Of course, you don't need a Belgian waffle maker to enjoy these, any type will do, but they are definitely better bigger! Top with your favorite toppings… I'm partial to Cherry Vanilla Compote or Sweetened Whipped Coconut Cream.

1 cup sorghum flour
½ cup superfine brown rice flour
¼ cup potato starch
¼ cup tapioca flour
1 teaspoon xanthan gum
4 tablespoons sugar
4 teaspoons baking powder
¾ teaspoon salt
2 tablespoons lemon juice
5 tablespoons olive oil
1 teaspoon vanilla extract
½ cup canned full-fat coconut milk
1½ cups water

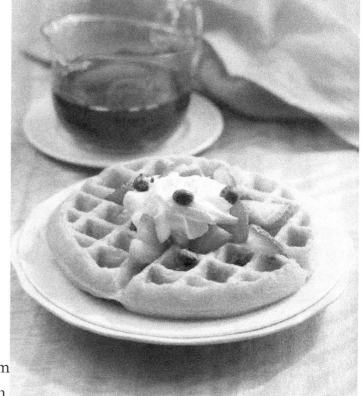

- In a medium bowl, whisk together the sorghum flour, superfine brown rice flour, potato starch, tapioca flour, xanthan gum, sugar, baking powder, and salt.

- Form a well in the center of the flour mixture and add the lemon juice, olive oil, vanilla extract, coconut milk, and water.

- Stir gently with a fork until all ingredients are combined, and then use a whisk to make the batter completely smooth.

- Heat your Belgian waffle maker and lightly mist with nonstick cooking spray. Pour about 1¼ cups batter (depending on your waffle maker's size) and close. Cook for about 2 minutes, or until waffle is golden brown and easily releases from the waffle iron.

APPLE FRITTERS

YIELD: 15 FRITTERS

Like pocket-size apple pies, these crunchy fritters are hard to resist! I love making these when I over purchase during apple season as this is a great recipe to get friends and family to gobble up all those extra apples quickly! You'll need a deep fryer for these to achieve a perfect crunch and quick, even cooking throughout.

3 apples, peeled
1 cup besan/chickpea flour, plus ½ cup for dredging
⅔ cup sugar
⅔ cup non dairy milk
½ teaspoon salt
½ teaspoon cinnamon Oil for frying
Turbinado and confectioner's sugar for dusting

- Preheat deep fryer to 360°F. Slice apples into ¼- to ½-inch-thick circles and use a small circular cookie cutter or apple corer to remove the seeds to form rings.

- In a medium-size bowl, whisk together the besan, sugar, non dairy milk, salt, and cinnamon until smooth. Once the fryer is ready, dredge the apple slices in the extra besan and then dip into the batter to completely coat.

- Fry apples three to four at a time for 5 minutes, flipping over two-thirds of the way through cooking time. Transfer to a paper towel– or paper bag– lined baking sheet (they will be soft at first) and then sprinkle with turbinado and confectioner's sugar. Repeat until all batter/apple slices have been fried.

- Let cool for at least 10 minutes before serving. Serve the same day, best within 1 hour of preparing.

STRAWBERRY TOASTER PASTRIES

YIELD: 6 PASTRIES

As a kid, I was obsessed with boxed toaster pastries, but, as I grew older and wiser about food, I became quite unimpressed with their extremely long ingredient lists. These pastries are just as tasty without the unpronounceable ingredients. You'll also find a brown sugar variation below.

FILLING

3 tablespoons strawberry jam

1½ teaspoons cornstarch mixed with

1½ teaspoons water

Dash salt

1 recipe Flakey Classic Piecrust

1 tablespoon flaxseed meal

2½ tablespoons water

- In a small bowl, combine the ingredients for the filling until smooth. Preheat oven to 350°F.

- Prepare the Flakey Classic Pie Crust according to recipe directions and chill for about 15 minutes in the freezer. Roll out in between two sheets of parchment paper until the dough is about ¼ inch thick. Use a pizza wheel or large flat knife to cut the dough into twelve even rectangles, about 3 × 4 inches wide; use a metal spatula to help transfer six of the rectangles to a parchment or silicone mat covered cookie sheet. Place the rectangles about 1 inch apart.

- Combine the flaxseed meal and water and let rest until thickened, for about 5 minutes. Lightly brush the tops of the rectangles on the cookie sheet with the flaxseed gel. Place about 1½ tablespoons filling into the center of the six rectangles. Use a spatula to help transfer the remaining six rectangles to cover each mound of filling.

- Crimp the sides of the dough to seal using the tines of a fork. Brush the tops lightly with additional flaxseed gel and poke about seven holes in the tops of each pastry. Bake for 30 to 35 minutes, or until golden brown on edges. Let cool completely and toast in toaster oven before serving. Top with Royal Icing or leave plain. Store in airtight container for up to 2 days.

BROWN SUGAR CINNAMON VARIATION

¼ cup brown sugar

½ teaspoon cinnamon

2 tablespoons brown rice flour

Whisk together the ingredients and use in place of the strawberry filling in the recipe. Top with Vanilla Glaze or Maple Glaze.

Chapter 5

FABULOUS FROZEN TREATS

Chill out with the cool treats on the following pages. Whether you're craving a sweet fix during the summertime, or you just need some fuel to help you veg out during a wintertime movie marathon, you'll be glad to have these recipes on hand (or in your freezer) when the craving strikes. You may be surprised that non dairy milks, such as almond, cashew, and coconut, do a remarkable job of replicating that creamy dreamy texture we crave from traditional-style ice cream. When choosing alternative milks for your ice cream, just like traditional ice cream, the higher the fat content the better!

Making Ice Cream Without a Machine

While it is possible to make ice cream without an ice cream machine, I do recommend sourcing an ice cream maker (from hand-crank to fully electric) if you make your own frequently, as I do. It is the best way to create unique flavors that are hard to come by in dairy-/egg-free versions at the supermarket or local gelataria.

I recommend using a machine only because of the amount of air that is able to be incorporated into the mix as it freezes, resulting in a lighter, airier texture, which is difficult to replicate without a machine. It is, however, easy to come pretty close. Most important, I recommend starting with a base that has a heavy fat content, such as the Vanilla Soft Serve or Chocolate Hazelnut Ice Cream. This will help reduce the odds of ice crystals forming while freezing, producing a smoother, creamier treat. Also, dropping a touch of alcohol (such as vodka or bourbon) into the mix, or using a recipe that incorporates alcohol before freezing will also help reduce crystallization.

Follow the directions for preparing your chosen recipe, and then place the mixture into a stainless steel or glass bowl and chill completely in the refrigerator, up to 8 hours. Whisk thoroughly to stir and then pour the mixture into a nonstick pan (plastic works well), stirring with a whisk after adding. Cover lightly with plastic wrap. Let the mixture chill in the freezer for 30 minutes, and then whisk again. You can incorporate more air by using an electric hand mixer for mixing. Chill for another 30 minutes, and then whisk (or blend) again. Repeat until the ice cream is frozen through and creamy. Transfer to a flexible airtight container. Most ice creams will last in the freezer for about 3 months.

ICE CREAM AND GELATO

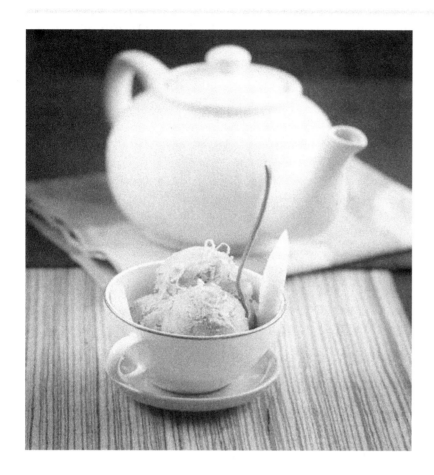

VANILLA SOFT SERVE

YIELD: 1 PINT

I absolutely adore flavors and add-ins of all kinds but, if I had to pick a favorite ice cream flavor, it wouldn't be anything fancy, just plain ol' vanilla. This ice cream is rich and dreamy and has a light vanilla flavor that lingers.

1 cup sugar

1 tablespoon agave

½ teaspoon xanthan gum

2 tablespoons vanilla extract

2 tablespoons coconut oil or non dairy margarine

1 cup non dairy milk (recommend almond or cashew)

1 cup canned full-fat coconut milk

- In a large bowl, whisk together the sugar, agave, xanthan gum, vanilla extract, coconut oil, and nondairy milk. Transfer to a blender and process until totally smooth. Whisk in the 1 cup coconut milk and process in an ice cream maker according to manufacturer's instructions or process according to the directions in this book. Once blended, store in airtight, flexible container and freeze at least 6 hours before serving. Keeps for up to 3 months frozen.

CHOCOLATE ESPRESSO ICE CREAM

YIELD: 1 QUART

This distinctive dessert is just like an indulgent drink at a coffee shop—so dark and creamy, it will have you requesting a doppio!

⅔ cup non dairy sour cream or plain yogurt
1 cup confectioners sugar
½ cup cocoa powder
2 teaspoons espresso powder
1 (13.5-ounce) can full-fat coconut milk
¼ teaspoon salt

- In a large bowl, whisk together all the ingredients until completely smooth and absolutely no lumps remain. Process in an ice cream maker according to manufacturer's instructions, or process according to the directions in this book. Transfer to a flexible airtight container and freeze at least 6 hours before serving. Keeps for up to 3 months frozen.

BUTTER PECAN ICE CREAM

YIELD: 1 QUART

When I think of Butter Pecan Ice Cream, I think of my father. I'm not sure if it was his favorite flavor, but we always seemed to have a carton of it in the freezer when I was growing up, which undoubtedly helped make it one of *my* favorite flavors of ice cream.

1 cup pecans
1 cup brown sugar
1 (13.5-ounce) can full-fat coconut milk
1 tablespoon non dairy margarine
¼ teaspoon xanthan gum
½ teaspoon salt
1 teaspoon vanilla extract
2 cups almond milk
1 tablespoon cornstarch
1 tablespoon water

- Preheat oven to 400°F. Spread the pecans evenly onto a metal baking sheet and toast for 7 minutes, or until fragrant. Let cool, chop, and set aside.

- In a 2-quart saucepan, whisk together the brown sugar, coconut milk, margarine, xanthan gum, salt, and vanilla extract. Heat the mixture over medium-high heat until the sugar is dissolved and the margarine is melted. Add the almond milk. In a small bowl, whisk together the cornstarch and water to mix well. Stir the cornstarch slurry into the saucepan and continue to heat over medium heat. Stir constantly until the mixture coats the back of a spoon. Remove from heat and transfer to a metal bowl. Place in refrigerator and chill the mixture until cold.

- Process in an ice cream maker according to manufacturer's instructions, or process according to the directions in this book. Once the ice cream is finished processing in the ice cream maker, fold in the toasted pecans. Transfer to a flexible airtight container and freeze for 6 hours. Store in the freezer for up to 2 months.

CHOCOLATE HAZELNUT ICE CREAM

YIELD: 1 PINT

Use store-bought or homemade chocolate hazelnut butter for this recipe.

½ cup non dairy chocolate hazelnut butter, such as Justin's brand
1 cup non dairy milk
2 tablespoons coconut oil
½ teaspoon xanthan gum
⅛ teaspoon salt
½ cup turbinado sugar
½ cup plain non dairy yogurt

- Place all the ingredients into a blender and blend until smooth, scraping the sides of the blender as needed. Process in your ice cream maker according to manufacturer's instructions or follow the directions in this book. Transfer to an airtight flexible container and store in freezer for at least 6 hours. Keeps for up to 3 months frozen.

BUTTERY BROWN SUGAR ICE CREAM

YIELD: 1 QUART

This ice cream proves you can have all of the indulgence of a buttery sweet flavor—without any of the dairy.

¼ cup non dairy margarine

1 cup brown sugar (light or dark)

½ teaspoon xanthan gum

1¾ cups canned full-fat coconut milk

½ teaspoon vanilla extract

⅔ cup non dairy milk

- Heat the margarine, brown sugar, xanthan gum, coconut milk, and vanilla extract just until sugar is dissolved and margarine is melted over medium heat. Stir in the nondairy milk and blend in blender. Chill for about 15 minutes, and then transfer into an ice cream maker. Following the manufacturer's instructions, process the ice cream until completely frozen, or process according to the directions in this book. Transfer to a flexible airtight container and chill in freezer for at least 6 hours. Store in the freezer for up to 3 months.

STRAWBERRY ICE CREAM

YIELD: 1 QUART

Forget the artificially flavored stuff, the only way to go with strawberry ice cream is with real strawberries! This is as authentic as you can get with the help of silken tofu and coconut milk to give it extra creaminess.

2 cups whole strawberries, stems removed
1 block (12.3 ounces) firm silken tofu
1 (13.5-ounce) can full-fat coconut milk 1 teaspoon vanilla extract
¾ cup sugar
1 teaspoon coconut oil
1 cup strawberries, chopped into ½-inch pieces

- Place the 2 cups strawberries into a blender along with the silken tofu, coconut milk, vanilla extract, sugar, and coconut oil. Blend until smooth and then transfer into the bowl of an ice cream maker and process according to manufacturer's instructions, or follow the method in this book. Once the mixture is mostly frozen, mash the remaining 1 cup strawberries and mix into the ice cream. Continue to process until frozen and then transfer to an airtight flexible container. Freeze 6 hours before serving. Keeps for up to 3 months frozen.

MATCHA CASHEW ICE CREAM

YIELD: 1 QUART

The magical cashew is the stand-in for traditional heavy whipping cream in this creamy confection. Matcha green tea powder adds a distinctive color and flavor, which matches the mellow texture of this ice cream.

2 cups raw cashews
½ cup agave
½ cup non dairy milk
¼ teaspoon salt
1½ teaspoons matcha powder
1 small ripe banana

• Place the cashews in a medium bowl and cover with water. Cap with a dinner plate and let the cashews soak for at least 3 hours, preferably 4.

• Drain the cashews and transfer into a food processor along with the remaining ingredients. Blend until very smooth, for about 8 minutes, scraping down the sides often. You can make this even creamier by transferring into a blender and blending until super smooth.

• Place in the bowl of an ice cream maker and process according to manufacturer's instructions, or follow directions in this book. Transfer to a flexible airtight container and freeze 6 hours before serving. Keeps for up to 3 months frozen.

MINT CHOCOLATE CHIP ICE CREAM

YIELD: 1 QUART

The brilliant green color of this dessert comes from the addition of fresh spinach, which I swear on my ice cream maker's life you won't taste. Make this even healthier by subbing cacao nibs in place of the mini chocolate chips.

2 cups packed fresh spinach
2 (13.5-ounce) cans full-fat coconut milk
½ cup sugar
½ cup coconut palm sugar
1 tablespoon agave
2 teaspoons peppermint extract
½ cup mini non dairy chocolate chips

Place all ingredients up to the chocolate chips into high-speed blender and blend until very smooth, scraping sides as needed. Pour into the bowl of an ice cream maker and process according to manufacturer's instructions, or follow the directions in this book. Once frozen, fold in the chocolate chips and freeze for at least 6 hours. Store in an airtight flexible container in the freezer for up to 3 months.

BLACK BEAN ICE CREAM

YIELD: 1 QUART

Adzuki beans work well here, too, although they can be harder to source.

1½ cups cooked black beans, rinsed
1 (13.5-ounce) can full-fat coconut milk
¾ cup sugar
1 tablespoon cocoa powder
Pinch of salt
⅛ teaspoon xanthan gum

* In a blender, puree all ingredients until very smooth. Process in your ice cream maker according to manufacturer's instructions, or follow the directions in this book. Store in a flexible airtight container and freeze at least 6 hours before serving. Keeps for up to 3 months frozen.

PUMPKIN PATCH ICE CREAM

YIELD: 1 QUART

The first time I tasted pumpkin flavored ice cream was right after a hayride with my childhood bestie while we were in middle school. It was such a great memory, with the crisp fall chill in the evening breeze and the smell of leaves crunching underneath our feet. Now, each time I taste pumpkin ice cream, I get transported right back to that day, autumnal bliss and all.

1½ cups sugar

1 (13.5-ounce) can full-fat coconut milk

2 teaspoons vanilla extract

1 (15-ounce) can pumpkin puree

1½ teaspoons cinnamon

⅛ teaspoon ground nutmeg

⅛ teaspoon cloves

½ teaspoon salt

- Over medium heat, in a 2-quart saucepan, warm the sugar and coconut milk just until the sugar has completely dissolved. Whisk in the vanilla extract, pumpkin puree, spices, and salt. Process in an ice cream maker according to manufacturer's instructions, or follow the directions in this book. Transfer to a flexible airtight container and freeze at least 6 hours before serving. Store in freezer for up to 3 months.

CHOCOLATE EARL GREY GELATO

YIELD: 1 QUART

This popular flavor combination gets its time to shine in this recipe. The floral notes of Earl Grey are subtle, but unforgettable.

7 Earl Grey tea bags
¾ cup very hot water
1 cup non dairy chocolate chips
¾ cup sugar
1 (13.5-ounce) can full-fat coconut milk
1 tablespoon extra-dark cocoa powder
Dash salt
¼ teaspoon xanthan gum, optional, for creaminess
½ cup non dairy milk

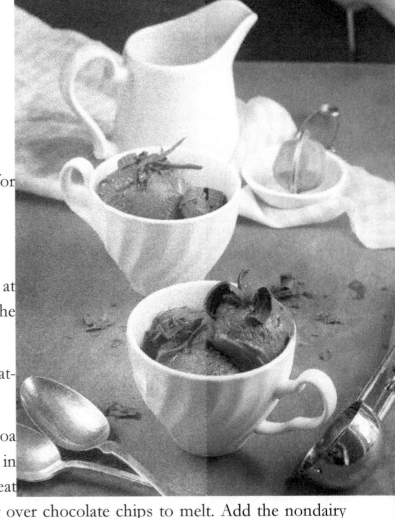

- Steep the tea bags in the hot water for at least 15 minutes. Squeeze and remove the tea bags and set tea aside.

- Place the chocolate chips in a large heat-safe bowl.

- Combine the sugar, coconut milk, cocoa powder, salt, and xanthan gum, if using, in a small saucepan over medium heat. Heat just until hot (do not let boil) and pour over chocolate chips to melt. Add the nondairy milk and prepared tea and stir well to combine. Chill the mixture in the refrigerator for 1 hour.

- Place into an ice cream maker and let run just until thickened to a soft serve ice cream consistency, or follow instructions in this book. Transfer immediately to a flexible airtight container and chill at least 6 hours until firm. Keeps for up to 3 months frozen.

BLACKBERRY CHEESECAKE GELATO

YIELD: 1 QUART

I dare you to take just one bite of this creamy concoction; the flavor is highly addictive. The bright purple hue that comes from the blackberries takes this gelato over the top. If blackberries aren't available, feel free to replace with another type of berry, frozen or fresh—all berries go great with cheesecake- flavored gelato! You can use Sweet Cashew Cream in place of the non dairy cream cheese if you like.

2 cups blackberries
1 cup non dairy cream cheese
1 cup non dairy milk
¾ cup sugar
1½ teaspoons vanilla extract

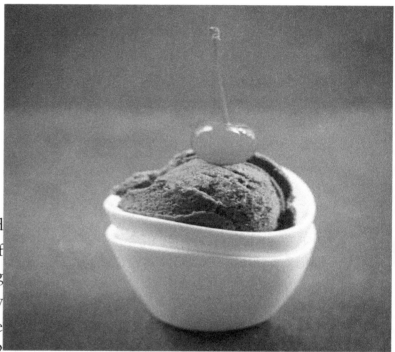

- Place all ingredients into a blender and blend until smooth. Transfer to the bowl of an ice cream maker and process according to manufacturer's directions, or follow directions in this book. Once frozen, store in a flexible airtight container for up to 2 months.

BUTTERSCOTCH PUDDING POPS

YIELD: 6 POPS

These pudding pops make the perfect warm weather treat with their salty butterscotch base and creamy cool texture. You'll need popsicle molds for these, or you can use silicone ice cube trays for mini-pops, or you can even use small paper cups.

1 recipe Butterscotch Sauce
1 (13.5-ounce) can full-fat coconut milk
2 tablespoons coconut palm sugar
⅛ teaspoon salt
3 tablespoons superfine brown rice flour

- In a 2-quart saucepan over medium heat, combine the Butterscotch Sauce, coconut milk, coconut palm sugar, and salt and whisk well until combined. Heat just until the mixture is hot and all coconut milk and sugar has dissolved. Whisk in the superfine brown rice flour and continue to cook over medium heat, stirring often, until thickened, for 4 to 5 minutes.

- Let cool briefly and then pour into popsicle molds, placing wooden sticks directly into the centers. Freeze overnight before enjoying. Keeps for up to 1 month frozen.

This recipe also makes a delicious Butterscotch Pudding—just don't freeze it! Instead, pour the pudding into serving dishes and refrigerate until set, for about 3 hours.

CLASSIC ICE CREAM SANDWICHES

YIELD: 8 SANDWICHES

This recipe produces a cookie that stands up well to freezing and stays soft once frozen, in a classic ice cream sandwich fashion. The base flavor is chocolate—pair the wafers with your favorite ice cream!

¾ cup cold non dairy margarine

1 cup sugar

1 teaspoon vanilla extract

1 cup sorghum flour

¾ cup cocoa powder

½ cup potato starch

1 teaspoon xanthan gum

¼ teaspoon baking soda

2 tablespoons non dairy milk

4 cups of your favorite non dairy ice cream

- In a large mixing bowl, cream together the margarine, sugar, and vanilla extract. In a separate, smaller mixing bowl mix the sorghum flour, cocoa powder, potato starch, xanthan gum, and baking soda until well combined.

- Gradually incorporate the flour mixture into the sugar mixture until crumbly. Once crumbly, add the non dairy milk until completely combined. If using an electric mixer, just let it ride on low as you add the non dairy milk. Your dough should get quite stiff at this point.

- Shape into a rectangular log, about 2 × 10 inches, using the help of parchment paper and a bench scraper/offset spatula to flatten and form the sides. Wrap loosely with parchment paper and chill in the freezer for 30 minutes, until very cold.

- Preheat oven to 350°F. Once the dough is well chilled, cut the log in half, making two even-sized bricks (about 2 × 5 inches each). Flip each brick on its side, and then slice evenly into rectangles about 2 × 3 inches and about
⅛ inch thick to emulate a cookie from a store-bought ice cream sandwich.

- As you slice the cookies, place each slab of thin dough gently onto parchment paper or a silpat mat.

213

- Bake in preheated oven for 14 to 16 minutes. Remove from oven and allow to cool completely at room temperature. Transfer to the freezer just before assembling and chill for at least 10 minutes. Meanwhile, soften your chosen ice cream for about 10 minutes, or until easily scoopable.

- To assemble, take one cookie, and plop a few spoonfuls of your favorite ice cream on top. Smoosh down the ice cream with another cookie and run a spoon around the edge to ensure even distribution of ice cream.

- Return sandwiches to freezer and chill until firm. Once firm, neatly wrap them in waxed paper to store. Keeps for up to 3 months frozen.

SORBETS AND ICES

ROSEMARY APPLE SORBET

YIELD: 1 QUART

I can't get enough of this sorbet. The apple flavor is really enticing and enhanced elegantly with the addition of rosemary. Be sure to seek out fresh rosemary, rather than dried, as it will absolutely make a difference.

2½ cups apple cider (no sugar added)
⅓ cup sugar
1 sprig fresh rosemary

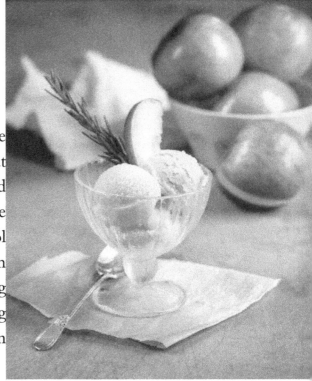

In a small saucepan over medium heat, combine the apple cider, sugar, and rosemary and cook for about 7 minutes, stirring often, until sugar is dissolved and the rosemary has added a hint of fragrance to the cider. Remove syrup from heat and let cool completely, either in the refrigerator, or at room temperature. Process in ice cream maker according to manufacturer's instructions or by following directions in this book. Once frozen, store in an airtight container in the freezer for up to 2 months.

STRAWBERRIES AND CHAMPAGNE SORBET

YIELD: 1 QUART

I don't actually recommend that you use Champagne to make this delightful sorbet, but you certainly can if you roll hard like that! I prefer Prosecco, for its subtle notes and its more modest price tag.

1 pear, peeled and cubed (about 1 cup)
2 cups strawberries, greens removed
1 cup Prosecco, Spumante, or other sparkling white wine
¾ cup sugar

- In a food processor, pulse together the pear and strawberries until well chopped. In a separate bowl, gradually mix the Prosecco with the sugar and stir gently to dissolve. Let rest for about 5 minutes and then stir gently again. Drizzle about ½ cup of the Prosecco mixture into the food processor and blend until quite smooth, for about 1 minute, scraping down the bowl as needed.

- Add in the rest of the Prosecco mixture and blend until very well combined. Transfer to the bowl of an ice cream maker and process according to manufacturer's instructions or by following directions on in this book.

- Store in an airtight container for up to 2 months in the freezer.

DRAGONFRUIT SORBET

YIELD: 1 QUART

Although I consider most all of nature's creations beautiful, I am always awestruck each time I cut into a dragonfruit. These bright fuchsia fruits open to a Dalmatian inside and have a neutral flavor similar to grapes. They make one heck of a gorgeous sorbet, too! Check for ripeness by gently pressing into the fruit's thick peel. If it gives to a little pressure under the thumb, then it's ripe.

2 large dragonfruits
1 cup sugar
1 cup water
¼ teaspoon vanilla extract

- Peel the dragonfruit by cutting the top stem section off just enough to reveal the white fruit. Gently peel the fruit as you would a banana to remove the skin cleanly and easily.

- Cube the fruit and place into a food processor. Pulse until the consistency of a slushy.

- In a small saucepan over medium heat, cook the sugar and water together just until the sugar has completely dissolved, for 1 to 2 minutes.

- Transfer the pureed dragonfruit into a bowl and mix in the sugar syrup and vanilla. Chill the mixture in the freezer for 30 minutes, stir, chill for 10 more minutes, then process in an ice cream maker until it is bright white and the consistency of sorbet. This can also be made following the directions in this book, but an ice cream maker is preferred if available. Store in flexible airtight container in freezer for up to 3 months.

GINGER PEACH SHERBET

YIELD: 1 QUART

Warm ginger combines so beautifully with this cool peach sherbet to bring a dessert that would be welcome at the end of any dinner party.

4 large ripe peaches (not too soft)
1 teaspoon fresh grated ginger
Dash salt
1 cup sugar
½ cup canned full-fat coconut cream (thickest part from a can of milk)
½ cup non dairy milk

- Fill a 2-quart pot about halfway with water and bring to a boil over medium-high heat. Carefully place peaches into the boiling water and cook for 1½ minutes. Drain immediately and gently run the peaches under cold water. Carefully remove the skins and pits and discard.

- Place the blanched peaches, ginger, salt, sugar, coconut cream, and nondairy milk into a food processor or blender and blend until smooth. Chill in the refrigerator until cold and then transfer to an ice cream maker and process according to manufacturer's instructions, or follow the directions in this book. Transfer to a flexible airtight freezable container and freeze for at least 4 hours before serving. Keeps for up to 3 months frozen.

STRAWBERRY BALSAMIC SORBETTO

YIELD: 2 CUPS

An absolutely delightful dessert, this tastes just like fresh-picked strawberries. The balsamic complements the berries well and counteracts the sweetness of the simple syrup.

¾ cup Simple Syrup
1 tablespoon white or red balsamic vinegar
2 cups fresh strawberries, greens removed

- In a blender, puree all the ingredients until smooth. Place in metal baking dish, about 8 inches round, and cover with plastic wrap. Freeze for 3 hours, or until solid, but still soft. Store in airtight container in freezer for up to 2 months.

LIMONCELLO SEMIFREDDO

YIELD: 6 SERVINGS

A bright and boozy treat that's for adults only. This creamy, fluffy, semifreddo is best made in a high-speed blender, such as a Vitamix, for extra airiness.

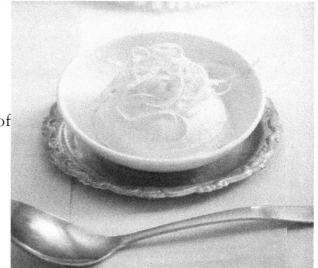

2 cups raw cashews
½ cup sugar
1 cup coconut cream (from the tops of 2 chilled cans of full-fat coconut milk)
⅔ cup Limoncello
Fresh lemon zest, for garnish (optional)

- Place the cashews into a medium bowl and cover with water. Let the cashews soak for least 4 hours, but no longer than 6. Drain and place into a high-speed blender.

- Add the rest of the ingredients and blend on low just to combine. Increase speed to high and let blend until completely smooth, for about 1 minute.

- Pour the mixture into silicone baking cups or ice cream molds and freeze for at least 6 hours and up to overnight. For an extra-special touch, serve garnished with lemon zest. Keeps for up to 3 months frozen.

ALMOND CHAMOMILE GRANITA

YIELD: ABOUT 3 CUPS

Such a soothing treat for a hot summer day, this light-tasting granita is a great choice when ice cream seems too heavy. The chamomile adds a floral note that's perfectly offset with the almond milk.

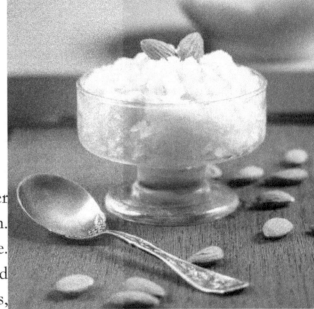

2 chamomile tea bags (or 2 teaspoons chamomile tea in tea strainer)
1 cup very hot, but not boiling, water
½ cup Simple Syrup
1 teaspoon almond extract
½ cup almond milk

- In a medium bowl, steep the tea and the hot water for 5 minutes, until the water is fragrant and golden. Remove tea bags and let cool to room temperature. Mix with the syrup, almond extract, and almond milk. Place in metal baking dish, about 8 × 8 inches, on flat surface in freezer. Chill mixture until frozen solid and then scrape into granules using a fork. Serve in chilled dishes. Keeps for up to 3 months frozen if stored in airtight container.

MOJITO GRANITA

YIELD: 3 CUPS

I love mojitos in the summertime. I get giddy when I see the fresh mint peek over our fence in the springtime, letting me know it's almost time to stock up on lime and seltzer. This granita will satisfy your craving for the summertime libation any time of year.

¾ cup Simple Syrup
Juice of 3 limes, about 6 tablespoons
2 tablespoons rum
1 cup cold sparkling water
½ teaspoon mint extract

- Combine all the ingredients in a medium bowl, and then pour into a nonstick plastic or metal dish. Freeze for 3 hours. Once frozen, gently scrape the mixture into granules using the tines of a fork. Serve with a fresh sprig of mint or a lime twist. Store in airtight container in the freezer. Keeps for up to 3 months frozen.

MANDARIN ICE

YIELD: 1 QUART

This delightful frozen treat is a refreshing way to get your vitamin C! I like using clementines, for extra sweetness, but tangerines or other oranges work nicely, too.

1½ cups mandarin juice, about 8 clementines' worth
2 teaspoons rum or vanilla extract
1 tablespoon agave

- Place all the ingredients into a bowl and whisk together well to combine. Pour into a metal cake pan (about 9 inches round) and place into the freezer. Freeze for 4 hours, or until frozen solid. Gently but quickly scrape the mixture into ice with a fork—don't overdo it or it may turn to a slushy— and then transfer into a sealable airtight container. Keeps for up to 3 months frozen.

PINEAPPLE ICE POPS

YIELD: ABOUT 4 POPS

These tropical treats are actually quite popular in Mexico and are referred to as *paleta de pina*. Paleta have countless flavor variations, but I love these pineapple pops because of the natural candy-like flavor of the pineapple.

You'll need popsicle molds or silicone ice cube trays for mini-pops or simply use small paper cups.

2 cups diced pineapple, drained
½ cup Simple Syrup
½ teaspoon rum or vanilla extract
2 tablespoons full-fat coconut milk

- Place all ingredients into a blender or food processor and blend until mostly pureed. Pour into popsicle molds, place wooden sticks into the center, and freeze overnight. Keeps for up to 3 months frozen.

Use agave in place of the simple syrup if desired, but expect a darker color to your pops.

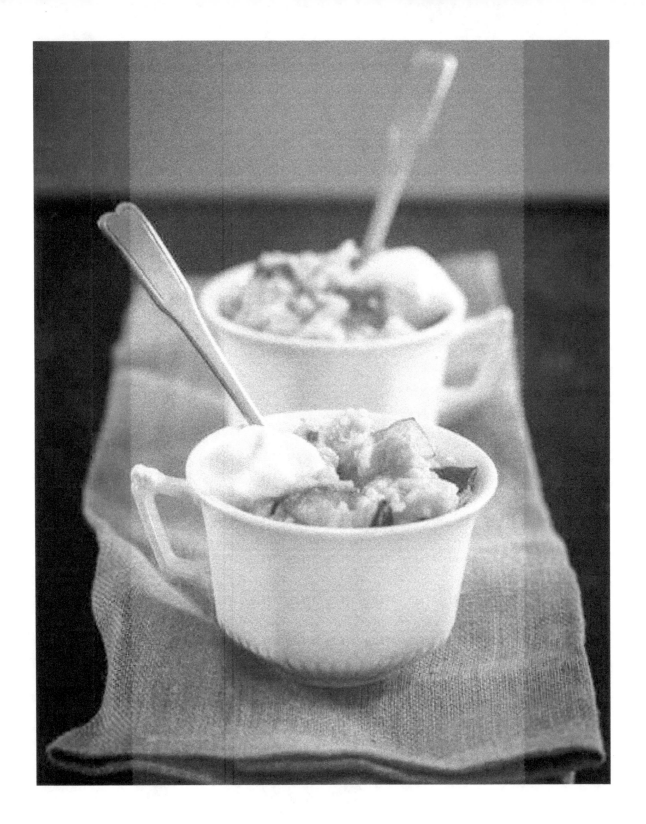

Chapter 6

TEMPTING PUDDINGS, CUSTARDS, JELLIES, AND FRUITS

This chapter covers everything you need to know for perfect puddings, fillings, fruits, and more. These are some of my favorite desserts to make because of the quickness and ease, as well as their uses in other desserts as fillings, toppings, and garnishes.

PUDDINGS AND CUSTARDS

CRÈME BRÛLÉE

YIELD: 4 SERVINGS

If you thought that getting just the right texture for classic crème brûlée would be impossible without eggs and cream, this recipe will prove just the opposite! If you don't have a culinary torch (why not?! … they're so much fun), then you can also place these under a broiler set on high for 5 minutes; just watch carefully so that you don't burn the sugar tops.

1 (13.5-ounce) can full-fat coconut milk
1½ cups non dairy milk
1 cup water 1¾ cups sugar
3 tablespoons non dairy margarine
¾ cup cornstarch mixed with ½ cup water
3 tablespoons besan/chickpea flour
1 teaspoon vanilla extract
¾ teaspoon sea salt
2 tablespoons sugar for topping

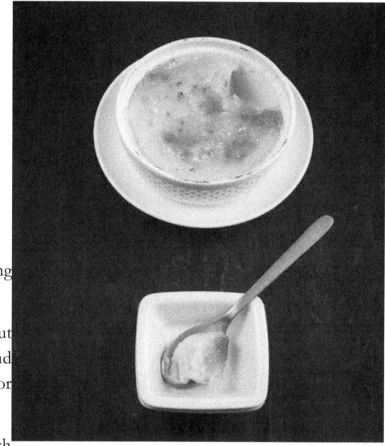

- Prepare four ramekins by very lightly greasing them with coconut oil or margarine.

- In a 2-quart saucepan, combine the coconut milk, non dairy milk, water, sugar, and margarine and cook over medium heat for about 5 minutes, or until the mixture is hot.

- In a small bowl, mix together the cornstarch slurry, besan, and vanilla extract until very smooth. Add the cornstarch mixture into the coconut milk mixture along with the salt and stir constantly with a whisk over medium heat to let it thicken, which should happen after about 5 minutes.

- Transfer to the prepared ramekins and let cool completely at room temperature until firm. Sprinkle each cup with about ½ tablespoon sugar, then brûlée the tops using a blowtorch. Store in airtight container for up to 1 week in refrigerator.

CHOCOLATE PUDDING

YIELD: 2 TO 4 SERVINGS

One of my favorite treats is chocolate pudding. I love how involved it all seems, standing over the stove, meditatively whisking away. This pudding is just as great as other Chocolate Puddings that we know and love with its thick and creamy texture and an unforgettably chocolate flavor.

½ cup cocoa powder

½ cup sugar

2 teaspoons vanilla extract

¼ teaspoon salt

1 cup non dairy milk

3 tablespoons cornstarch

3 tablespoons water

- In a 2-quart saucepan, whisk together the cocoa powder, sugar, vanilla extract, salt, and about ⅓ cup of the non dairy milk. Mix until very smooth with no lumps remaining, and then add in the additional non dairy milk.

- Warm over medium heat. In a small bowl, whisk together the cornstarch and water until no lumps remain. Stir in the cornstarch slurry and keep stirring continuously, over medium heat, until thickened, for about 5 minutes. Transfer to two medium or four small dishes and chill before serving. Store in airtight container for up to 1 week in refrigerator.

PISTACHIO PUDDING

YIELD: 2 TO 4 SERVINGS

This slightly salty and oh-so-sweet treat is easy to bring together and a sure winner for the pistachio lover in your life. I especially love this rich pudding served in small amounts as a dessert or aperitif.

1 cup roasted and salted pistachios, shelled
½ cup granulated sugar
⅓ cup non dairy milk, plus 1½ cups non dairy milk
¼ cup additional granulated sugar
5 tablespoons cornstarch
4 tablespoons water

- In a food processor, pulse the pistachios until crumbly. Add in sugar and blend until powdery—with just a few larger chunks remaining. Add the ⅓ cup nondairy milk and puree until very well combined.

- Transfer pistachio mixture to a 2-quart pot and whisk in the additional nondairy milk and sugar.

- In a small bowl, use a fork to combine the cornstarch and water until no lumps remain. Add this slurry to the pistachio mixture.

- Heat over medium heat, stirring frequently until thickened, for 5 to 7 minutes. Pour into two to four ramekins or serving dishes and let cool completely. Serve chilled with whipped topping! Store in airtight container for up to 1 week in refrigerator.

VANILLA PLUM RICE PUDDING

YIELD: 6 SERVINGS

A fragrant take on traditional rice pudding, I like to use basmati for its gorgeous floral notes in addition to the vanilla and plum.

¾ cup basmati or long-grain rice
1½ cups cold water
3 plums, unpeeled, stone removed, and diced
3 teaspoons vanilla extract
½ teaspoon salt
1 cup non dairy milk
½ cup sugar
2 tablespoons sweet white rice flour
¼ cup water

- In a 2- or 3-quart saucepan with a tight-fitting lid, stir together the rice and the cold water. Bring to a boil over medium-high heat. Immediately reduce to a simmer and cover. Do not stir.

- Let simmer for about 20 minutes, or until rice can be fluffed easily with a fork. Increase heat to medium and stir in the plums, vanilla extract, salt, nondairy milk, and sugar. In a smaller bowl, use a fork to stir together the sweet white rice flour and water. Stir the slurry into the rice mixture and cook for about 5 to 7 minutes, stirring constantly, until thick. Serve warm or cold. Store in airtight container for up to 1 week in refrigerator.

TAPIOCA PUDDING

YIELD: 6 SERVINGS

Tapioca pudding is one of those desserts that most people either love or hate, and I truly do adore it! Having grown up with only the instant puddings, I find this homemade version is so much better. It may change your mind if you're not a fan already. Seek out tapioca pearls in the baking section of most grocery stores, or find an endless variety of shapes and colors in Asian markets.

½ cup small tapioca pearls (not instant)
1 cup canned full-fat coconut milk
2 cups non dairy milk
½ teaspoon salt
½ cup sugar
1 teaspoon vanilla

- In a 2-quart pot, whisk together all the ingredients until smooth. Over medium-high heat, bring to a boil, stirring constantly. Once boiling, reduce heat to low and simmer for 15 minutes, stirring very often, until pudding is thickened and pearls are no longer white and firm but instead clear and gelatinous.

- Place into serving dishes or a flexible airtight container and chill until completely cold. Serve cold. Store in airtight container for up to 1 week in refrigerator.

FALL HARVEST QUINOA PUDDING

YIELD: 6 SERVINGS

Fruits and fall-time spices combine to make one comforting pudding, and the quinoa gives it a dense, creamy, and chewy texture.

1 tablespoon coconut oil
1 cup chopped pecan pieces
1 apple, chopped into small pieces
½ cup dried dates, chopped
½ teaspoon ground nutmeg
1 teaspoon ground cinnamon
¼ teaspoon cardamom
½ teaspoon salt
½ cup cold non dairy milk
2 teaspoons cornstarch
1 teaspoon vanilla extract
2 cups cooked quinoa
1 cup brown sugar

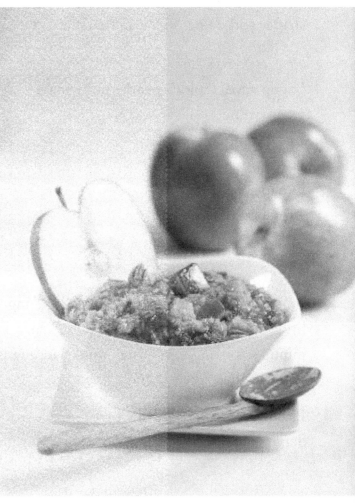

- Over medium heat, in a 2-quart saucepan, warm the coconut oil until melted. Add the pecans, apples, dates, nutmeg, cinnamon, cardamom, and salt. Continue to cook over medium heat, stirring as to not let the mixture burn. Cook for 3 to 5 minutes, or until apples soften and pecans become fragrant.

- In a small bowl, mix the non dairy milk with the cornstarch and vanilla extract. Whisk together until well combined and no lumps are visible.

- Add the cooked quinoa to the saucepan. Stir in the brown sugar and nondairy milk mixture. Cook over medium heat for about 2 minutes, or until thickened. Serve warm or chilled. Store in airtight container for up to 1 week in refrigerator.

PUMPKIN FLAN

YIELD: 4 SERVINGS

This is a traditional method of making pumpkin flan, where the pumpkin is allowed to shine on its own, rather than being masked by spices like cinnamon and cloves.

1 cup canned pumpkin or strained pumpkin puree
1 cup non dairy milk
½ cup + 1 tablespoon sugar
¼ teaspoon salt
Dash ground nutmeg
⅓ cup cornstarch
4 tablespoons cold water

- Lightly grease four ramekins or teacups with margarine or cooking spray.

- In a 2-quart saucepan, whisk together the pumpkin, non dairy milk, sugar, salt, and nutmeg until smooth. Warm over medium heat.

- Combine the cornstarch with the cold water and stir until no lumps remain. Drizzle into the pumpkin mixture and continue to whisk, constantly, over medium heat until thickened, for about 7 minutes. You will notice a significant strain on your wrist as it becomes thickened.

- Pour/spoon into lightly greased ramekins and let cool. Transfer to refrigerator and chill completely until cold. Invert onto a small flat plate, or leave in cups for serving. Top with Caramel Sauce. Store in airtight container for up to 1 week in refrigerator.

CREAMSICLE CUSTARD

YIELD: 4 SERVINGS

This pudding's sunny orange flavor will brighten your day. You can even freeze this pudding in popsicle molds to make creamsicles!

4 tablespoons cornstarch
4 tablespoons cold water
2 cups non dairy milk
½ cup freshly squeezed orange juice
1 cup sugar
1 teaspoon orange zest
½ teaspoon salt

- In small bowl whisk together the cornstarch and cold water and mix well until dissolved. In a small saucepan, combine the non dairy milk, orange juice, and sugar. Stir in the zest and salt. Warm up slightly over medium- low heat, and gradually add in the cornstarch slurry while stirring frequently with a whisk until the mixture reaches a slow boil.

- Reduce heat to low and continue to stir until the mixture becomes thick, for about 10 minutes cooking time total. Divide between four serving dishes and let sit at room temperature until warm. Transfer the dishes to the refrigerator and chill for at least 3 hours, or until it is completely set. Serve chilled. Store in airtight container for up to 1 week in refrigerator.

TIRAMISU

YIELD: 10 SERVINGS

Tiramisu is perhaps one of the most popular desserts at Italian restaurants. I always love Tiramisu for its intoxicating fragrance and delightfully melt-in- your-mouth texture. After going gluten-free, I was convinced this dessert would be off limits for good, but no more! Allergy-friendly fancy dessert, at your service.

10 to 12 Ladyfingers

¼ recipe Devilishly Dark Chocolate Sauce

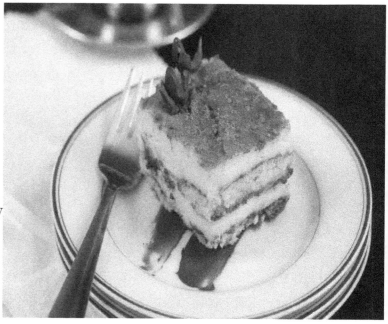

FILLING

1 recipe Mascarpone

1½ cups confectioner's sugar

⅛ teaspoon salt

12 ounces firm silken tofu

3 ounces (about 3 tablespoons) non dairy cream cheese

3 tablespoons cornstarch

4 tablespoons cold water

SAUCE

1 tablespoon cocoa powder, plus more for dusting

1 tablespoon agave

2 tablespoons very strong coffee or espresso

For the Filling

- Place the Mascarpone, confectioner's sugar, salt, tofu, and nondairy cream cheese into a food processor and blend until very smooth, for about 2 minutes. Transfer the mixture into a 2-quart saucepan over medium heat.

- Whisk together the cornstarch and cold water until no lumps remain. Drizzle the cornstarch slurry into the rest of the ingredients and whisk together, continuing to cook over medium heat. Keep stirring continuously until the mixture thickens, for about 5 minutes. Do not walk away from the mixture or it will burn!

- Let cool briefly.

For the Sauce

- Prepare the sauce by whisking together the cocoa powder, agave, and coffee in a small bowl until smooth.

To assemble the Tiramisu

- In a small, square baking pan, arrange five or six ladyfinger cookies to fit into the pan. Spread the Cocoa Espresso Sauce into a shallow flat dish, big enough for the cookies to lay flat. One by one, dip each side of the cookie into the sauce, briefly, and carefully replace. Repeat until all the cookies have been lightly dipped.

- Divide the Tiramisu filling in half and spread half of the filling on top of the ladyfingers and repeat with one more layer of each. Dust the top with cocoa powder and then drizzle with the Devilishy Dark Chocolate Sauce right before serving. Store in airtight container for up to 3 days in refrigerator.

BROWNIE BATTER MOUSSE

YIELD: 6 SERVINGS

Tiny bites of chocolate-covered walnuts—that taste a heck of a lot like miniature brownies—speckle this silky mousse, delivering a double dose of chocolate flavor.

6 ounces chopped semi-sweet chocolate

2 tablespoons non dairy milk

1 tablespoon maple syrup

1 cup roughly chopped walnuts

2 (350 g) packages extra-firm silken tofu

1 cup sugar

¾ cup cocoa powder

½ teaspoon salt

1 teaspoon vanilla extract

- Melt the chocolate in a double boiler over low heat until smooth. Stir in the nondairy milk and maple syrup and remove from the heat. Add the walnuts and coat liberally with a thick chocolate layer.

- Line a cookie sheet with a silicone mat or waxed paper. Spread the chocolate-covered walnuts in an even layer on the prepared cookie sheet. Chill the walnuts in your freezer until you are finished making the mousse.

- To make the mousse, simply blend the tofu, sugar, cocoa powder, salt, and vanilla extract in a food processor or blender until extremely smooth, for about 2 minutes, scraping down the sides as needed.

- Remove the chocolate-covered walnuts from the freezer when they are firm and stir them into the mousse. Spoon into individual dishes and serve very cold. Store in airtight container for up to 1 week in refrigerator.

BUTTERNUT POTS DE CRÈME

YIELD: 2 SERVINGS

Tender butternut squash is the base for this incredibly rich chocolate dessert. This makes a fabulous fall-time indulgence. The Pots de Crème can be made up to two days in advance.

2 cups cubed, roasted butternut squash
½ cup coconut sugar or packed brown sugar
¼ cup cocoa powder
¼ cup sorghum flour
1 teaspoon vanilla extract
½ teaspoon salt
Smoked salt for topping

- Preheat oven to 350°F and lightly grease two 4-inch ramekins.

- Puree the squash in food processor until smooth. Add in the sugar, cocoa powder, sorghum flour, vanilla extract, and salt. Blend until all ingredients are well combined, scraping the sides as needed.

- Spoon the mixture into the two ramekins and sprinkle smoked salt onto the custards. Bake for 45 to 50 minutes, or until the sides of the pudding begin to pull away from the ramekins. Serve hot for a softer pudding or serve chilled for a firm dessert. Store in airtight container for up to 1 week in refrigerator.

CHOCOLATE SOUP

YIELD: 4 SERVINGS

Somewhere in between pudding and chocolate sauce, this unusual dessert is such a fun choice for dinner parties. Serve this extra-rich dish in very small bowls.

1 cup canned coconut milk, lite or full-fat

¾ cup non dairy milk (unsweetened)

2 teaspoons vanilla extract

⅓ cup sugar

⅛ teaspoon salt

1 tablespoon cocoa powder

½ cup non dairy chocolate, chopped

1 tablespoon cornstarch mixed with 2 tablespoons water

- In a small saucepan, whisk together the coconut milk, non dairy milk, vanilla extract, sugar, salt, and cocoa powder. Heat over medium heat until very hot, but not yet boiling, for about 5 minutes. Stir in the chocolate, and heat just until melted, stirring continuously, making sure not to let the mixture come to a boil. Whisk in the cornstarch slurry and heat for about 3 minutes, stirring constantly, until the mixture has thickened and it coats the back of a spoon. Serve hot in individual bowls garnished with vegan marshmallows or Sweetened Whipped Coconut Cream and cacao nibs (or mini chocolate chips). Store in airtight container for up to 2 days in refrigerator. Reheat simply by warming over medium-low heat in small saucepan until desired temperature is reached.

BREAD PUDDING

YIELD: 8 SERVINGS

This pudding lends itself perfectly to mix-ins of all sorts. Try pineapple chunks mixed in and then top with toasted coconut for a tropical twist. Or, try mixing in chunks of a banana and ½ cup chocolate chips.

8 slices gluten-free bread
2 tablespoons melted non dairy margarine
¾ cup besan/chickpea flour
1½ cups non dairy milk
⅔ cup light brown sugar
1 teaspoon cinnamon
1 teaspoon vanilla extract
¼ cup raisins, or other dried fruit (optional)

- Preheat oven to 350°F and lightly grease an 8 × 8-inch baking pan.

- Cube the bread into bite-size pieces and arrange them evenly into the pan. Drizzle the bread with the melted margarine.

- In a small bowl, whisk together the besan, nondairy milk, brown sugar, cinnamon, and vanilla extract until no lumps remain in the batter.

- Pour the mixture evenly over the bread until it is fully covered. Press down on the bread pieces gently to fully submerge the bread in the batter. Sprinkle with raisins, if using.

- Bake for 35 to 40 minutes, or until golden brown on top and cooked through the center. Store in airtight container for up to 1 week in refrigerator. Reheat at 350°F for 10 minutes before serving.

CHOCOLATE BERRY PARFAITS

YIELD: 4 PARFAITS

These luscious parfaits are the perfect blend of tart and sweet, with just a touch of crunch from the cacao nibs. This makes a lovely treat for Valentine's Day, or just about any day!

1 cup red raspberries
2 cups strawberries, sliced
1 cup non dairy chocolate chips
12.3 ounces (349 g) extra-firm silken tofu
1 tablespoon agave
1 teaspoon vanilla extract
½ cup cacao nibs
½ cup Sweet Cashew Cream

- Toss the raspberries and strawberries together into a small bowl.

- Over a double boiler, melt your chocolate chips until very smooth. In a food processor, blend the silken tofu with the agave and vanilla extract. While the food processor is spinning, drizzle in your melted chocolate until all is combined.

- Assemble parfaits by layering in four fancy glasses the berries, cacao nibs, pudding, more berries, and more pudding, then top each glass with a dollop of Sweet Cashew Cream.

- Serve chilled. Store in airtight container for up to 1 week in refrigerator.

JELLIES, FRUITS, AND SAUCES

BELLINI GELEE

YIELD: 4 SERVINGS

This boozy dessert has all the crisp sweet flavor of the adult drink! Agar is used as a gelatin substitute in this gelled dessert. Be sure to dissolve the powder all the way or it won't set correctly.

1 cup peaches, blanched and pureed, or 1 cup peach nectar
1 cup sugar
3 cups Prosecco or Pinot Grigio
1 cup water
4 teaspoons agar powder

- Gather four sturdy wine glasses or medium silicone molds.

- Whisk together the pureed peaches, sugar, Prosecco, water, and agar in a 2- or 3-quart heavy saucepan. Bring to a boil, and then immediately reduce heat to low. Stir regularly and let simmer for 5 to 6 minutes.

- Let cool slightly, for about 10 minutes, before pouring into wine or champagne glasses or silicone molds.

- If you are using the silicone mold, be sure to place a larger, sturdier pan underneath the mold before you pour your liquid in, ensuring a smooth transport to the fridge.

- Let the mixture chill in the refrigerator until firm, for at least 2 hours. Store in airtight container for up to 1 week in refrigerator.

CRANBERRY FAUX-GURT

YIELD: 2 SERVINGS

The tart cranberries give this delectable treat an authentic yogurt flavor without the waiting. Top with fresh fruit and granola for an irresistible treat.

1 cup fresh cranberries
½ cup sugar or agave
1 tablespoon water
1 cup Sweet Cashew Cream
½ cup coconut cream (from the top of a can of coconut milk)

- In a small saucepan, over medium-low heat, cook the cranberries, sugar, and water until cranberries are very soft, for about 10 minutes. Let cool briefly and then blend in a blender along with the cashew cream and coconut cream until fluffy. Pour into jar and chill; mixture will thicken slightly upon chilling. Store in airtight container for up to 1 week in refrigerator.

CARAMEL ROASTED PEARS

YIELD: 4 SERVINGS

This is a simple recipe, but full of complex flavor.

4 red pears, peeled but stems left intact
⅓ cup agave
⅓ cup brown sugar or coconut sugar
2 tablespoons non dairy margarine, melted
⅓ cup canned coconut milk

- Preheat oven to 400°F. Carefully slice the bottoms of the pears straight across just to remove the nodule on the bottom, so that they easily stand in a small stoneware or metal baking dish.

- In a small bowl, mix together the agave, brown sugar, margarine, and coconut milk. Drizzle generously over the pears, and then allow the rest to fall to the bottom of baking dish. Bake in a preheated oven for 25 to 30 minutes, stopping to baste with the caramel sauce every 5 minutes or so, until the pears are tender and lightly golden brown.

- Carefully transfer using a flat metal spatula to a saucer or lipped dish with the sauce drizzled onto the pears. Serve immediately. Store leftovers in an airtight container in the refrigerator for up to 2 days.

THAI MANGO STICKY RICE

YIELD: 2 SERVINGS

One of my favorite parts about visiting a Thai restaurant is enjoying the Mango Sticky Rice when mangoes are in season. Luckily, this addictive treat can be made at home! When making this recipe, it's important to seek out "glutinous" rice, usually sold as "short grain" or "sticky" rice, which refers to the glue-like stickiness of the rice, not gluten.

1 cup short-grain glutinous rice

1½ cups canned full-fat coconut milk

1 cup water

3 tablespoons sugar

Dash salt

1 mango, peeled and sliced into strips

SAUCE
½ cup canned full-fat coconut milk

1½ tablespoons sugar

1 teaspoon cornstarch

2 teaspoons water

Dash salt

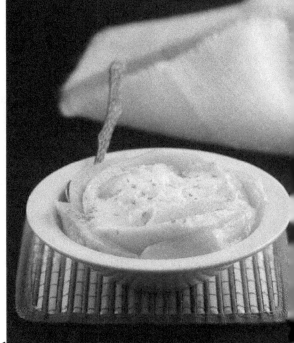

- Soak 1 cup rice in 3 cups of water for 1 hour. Drain and rinse the rice and place into a saucepan with a tight-fitting lid. Stir in coconut milk, water, sugar, and salt, and bring to a boil over medium-high heat. Once it hits a boil, immediately reduce the temperature to low, stir, cover, and simmer for about 20 minutes, or until all liquid is absorbed and rice is tender.

- To make the sauce, in a small saucepan, combine the coconut milk with the sugar. In a small bowl, whisk together the cornstarch and water until smooth. Whisk the cornstarch slurry and the salt into the coconut milk mixture and cook over medium heat, stirring constantly, until thickened.

- Plate by placing a small mound of cooked rice in a bowl, along with the sliced mangos, and top with the coconut sauce. Serve immediately.

BROILED PERSIMMONS

YIELD: 6 SERVINGS

If you've never had persimmons, you're in for a treat. This simple dish showcases the soft texture and almost peachy flavor of the fruit. Seek out persimmons between the months of October and February. Ripe persimmons will have bright orange, shiny skin and will be soft to the touch. You don't want to try and eat an unripe persimmon, as it will taste extremely chalky and unpleasant. A good test for ripeness lies in the calyx, or center tuft on top of the fruit: it will stay intact until ripened; once ripe, it can be easily removed from the fruit. To speed ripening, place in a paper bag in a dry place.

3 ripe persimmons, any variety
2 tablespoons agave
1 teaspoon vanilla extract
½ teaspoon lemon juice

- Preheat oven to broil.

- Slice the persimmons in half horizontally and place each, middle side up, so that they fit snugly into a ceramic or metal baking dish. In a small bowl, whisk together the agave, vanilla extract, and lemon juice and then brush the mixture liberally onto the tops of the persimmon halves.

- Broil for 8 to 10 minutes, rotating the pan at least once while cooking to evenly brown the fruits. Keep an eye on them so they do not burn, and broil just until browned evenly. Serve with Vanilla Soft Serve or Mascarpone. Serve immediately.

BAKED APPLES

YIELD: 6 SERVINGS

A warm and welcome treat come autumn, these are quick to make and fun to eat. I like to peel the apples so that I leave a stripe of peel for color. This works especially nicely with red apples, but green is pretty, too.

6 firm, tart apples such as Gala, Granny Smith, or Honeycrisp

FILLING

⅔ cup crushed walnuts (pulsed in food processor until crumbly)

⅔ cup certified gluten-free oats

2 tablespoons coconut oil

2½ tablespoons coconut palm sugar

¼ teaspoon cardamom

½ teaspoon cinnamon

Dash sea salt

½ cup golden raisins

- Core the apples making sure to leave the bottom intact. The easiest way to do this is to start with an apple corer and then use a small paring knife or vegetable peeler to scoop out a larger cavity to hold the filling.

- Next, peel the apples. Peel them only halfway, making a swirled design from the remaining skin.

- In a small bowl, combine the filling ingredients with a spoon until very well mixed. Stuff the apples with the filling, dividing evenly among the six apples.

- Preheat oven to 375°F and place the apples individually into a large-size muffin pan. Add 1 tablespoon water to the bottom of each muffin tin and then cover loosely with aluminum foil. Bake the apples for 35 to 40 minutes, or until apples are tender—don't overcook, or they will fall apart.

- Let cool briefly and then serve.

CHERRY VANILLA COMPOTE

YIELD: 2 CUPS

This recipe makes a delightful condiment and can be used in both sweet and savory combinations. I love the Chocolate Soup with a dollop of this compote in the center, along with a touch of Sweetened Whipped Coconut Cream.

2½ cups cherries, pitted
¼ cup coconut palm sugar
1 vanilla bean or 2 teaspoons vanilla extract
1 tablespoon brandy or rum

- In a heavy 2-quart saucepan, combine all the ingredients and, over medium heat, bring to a boil, while stirring often. Reduce the heat to medium low and cook for about 10 minutes, until cherries are soft.

- Strain the cherries, reserving the liquid. Pour the liquid back into the saucepan and simmer over medium-low heat until sauce is thickened, stirring occasionally, for about 15 to 20 minutes. Place cherries back into the syrup and serve warm. Store in airtight container for up to 1 week in refrigerator.

BLUEBERRY LAVENDER JAM

YIELD: 2½ CUPS

I especially love this stirred into some plain non dairy yogurt or chia pudding, and it even works well as a cheesecake topping.

1½ cups sugar
2 tablespoons fresh or dried lavender buds
¼ cup water
6 cups blueberries

- In a small saucepan, whisk together ½ cup of the sugar, lavender buds, and water. Simmer for 2 minutes, until fragrant, and then strain to remove the lavender buds. Transfer the scented sugar syrup along with the blueberries and remaining sugar into a 2-quart saucepan.

- Using a potato masher, gently smash the blueberries and cook over medium heat for 15 minutes. Let cool completely before transferring to jars. Store in sealed jars in refrigerator for up to 1 month.

The syrup used to make the preserves also makes a delicious addition to lemonade. Use the syrup in place of sugar and add lemon juice and water to taste. Store in airtight container for up to 1 week in refrigerator.

STRAWBERRY PRESERVES

YIELD: 2½ CUPS

I find myself using this type of preserve more than any other to add a touch of sweetness or flavor to many desserts. The amount of sugar in this recipe is essential in making the correct consistency; otherwise you may end up with a runny end result.

1 pound strawberries
2 cups sugar
2 tablespoons lemon juice

- Slice the strawberries and reserve the greens for another use, such as smoothies or salad greens.

- Place the fruit into a stockpot and combine with the sugar and lemon juice and heat over low heat just until the sugar is dissolved. Increase temperature to medium-high heat and bring the mixture to a boil, stirring constantly. Heat until the mixture registers 220°F on a candy thermometer.

- Transfer into sterile jars (a wash and dry on high heat through the dishwasher does the trick) and let cool to room temperature. Transfer to freezer, or, if you plan to eat right away, store in refrigerator in a sealed airtight jar for up to 2 weeks.

This jam as well as the Blueberry Lavender Jam and Cherry Vanilla Compote can certainly be processed in a water bath rather than transferred into a freezer.

QUICK AND EASY APPLESAUCE

YIELD: 6 CUPS

Applesauce is so easy to make, you really should give it a whirl if you never have. You may wonder why it has taken so long to DIY!

10 medium Granny Smith apples, peeled, cored, and sliced (about 11 cups)
¼ cup sugar (optional)
½ cup apple cider (or water)
2 teaspoons lemon juice

- In the bowl of a large slow cooker, toss together the apples and sugar. Mix together the apple cider and lemon juice and drizzle over the apples. Cover and cook on high for 3 hours, until very soft, stirring occasionally. Alternatively, cook for 6 hours on low temperature until very soft and completely transformed to applesauce. Store in airtight container for up to 1 week in refrigerator.

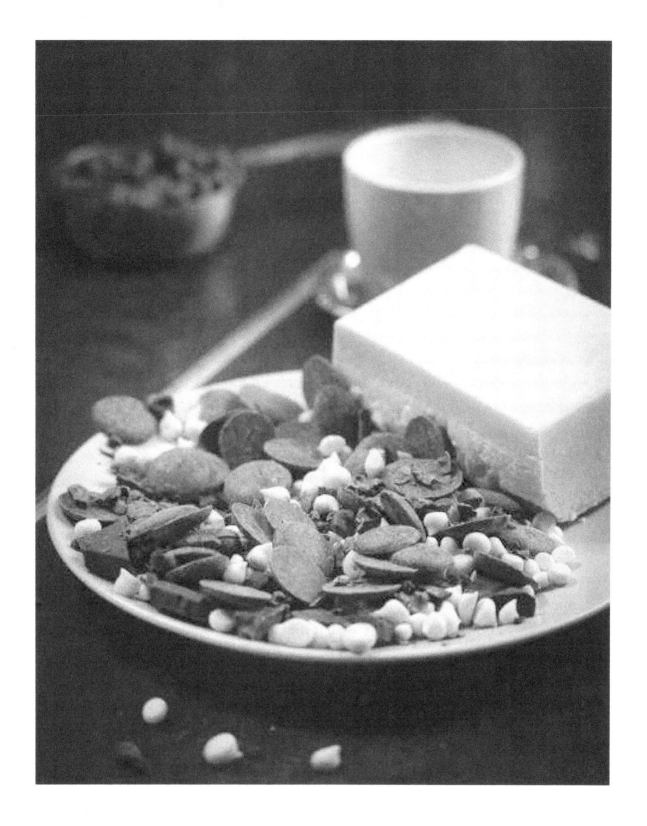

Chapter 7

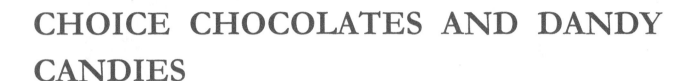

CHOICE CHOCOLATES AND DANDY CANDIES

Any candy craving can easily be satisfied at home once you get the knack for candy making—all it takes is a little patience and practice for results that far surpass store-bought. Plus, you can customize it! I've been making candy since I was tall enough to use the stove; so if you've never made candy before, don't be intimidated—even a child can do it! In this chapter you'll find recipes for everything from hard candies to chocolate treats to gooey chewy caramels.

CANDY MAKING BASICS

The best piece of advice I can give for making candy is to have all ingredients out and ready to go before beginning, and make sure you read the candy recipe instructions at least three times before beginning, until you have a clear grasp of how the recipe will work. The tricky thing about candy making is that it all happens so quickly once the sugar comes to the correct temperature, so you need to be prepared!

In the following recipes, be sure to follow the steps precisely. I recommend a (calibrated) candy thermometer for recipes requiring one, but, if you don't have one, you can always use the Cold Water Method. This is actually how I learned to make candy, so again, a very easy method that just takes a little practice to master.

COLD WATER METHOD

Place cup of ice-cold water next to your saucepan containing your candy mixture. Test for the candy doneness by dropping about a teaspoon or so of the hot syrup from a spoon into the cold water. Follow the temperature guidelines below, which outline the properties of the candy at each stage of doneness

Soft-Ball Stage

235°F–240°F

A soft, flexible ball that will flatten when removed from water.

Firm-Ball Stage

245°F–250°F

A firm ball that will hold its shape when removed from the water but is malleable.

Hard-Ball Stage

250°F–265°F

A firm ball that is a little more difficult to change the shape, but possible.

Soft-Crack Stage

270°F–290°F

Flexible threads will form when dropped into ice-cold water.

Hard-Crack Stage

300°F–310°F

This is the hottest stage of most candy recipes, so be sure to let the dropped syrup cool completely in the water before touching it in this stage. When sugar is dropped into the cold water, brittle hard threads will form.

WASH DOWN

When cooking sugar into candy, be sure to wash down the sugar crystals from the sides of the pan as you go. You can do this simply with a silicone brush dipped in a running stream of water. Just brush lightly over the crystals, as many times as needed, until all crystals are dissolved. This is important as a single sugar crystal can cause recrystallization, ruining the whole batch of candy. Always have a silicone or bristle brush handy to wash down the sides of your saucepan.

SAUCEPAN

When making candy it is important that you use a good-quality saucepan for best heat distribution. Too thin of a saucepan can cause scorching and other unpleasantries. You don't need to spend a lot of money, though; one of my favorite candy-making pots is an old Revere Ware copper-bottomed 3-quart pan that I learned to make candy with as a kid. It still serves me well today. I recommend a 2- or 3-quart pan for all the recipes listed, unless otherwise specified. Also, make sure that the sides of the pan are straight, so that you can get an accurate read on your thermometer.

CHOCOLATE BASICS

CHOOSING QUALITY CHOCOLATE

When you're out perusing the specialty food stores or hobby shops, you may notice that there are basically two different types of chocolate to choose from: couverture and baking chips, such as Ghirardelli. Couverture is very high quality chocolate that contains extra cocoa butter. You may be unable to find good-quality couverture at a supermarket but seek it out at specialty groceries, craft stores, or even online. Amazon has a good selection of dairy-free couverture at excellent prices.

The main difference between couverture and baking chips is the final outcome of the chocolate. Couverture results in a snappy, shiny texture (like chocolates from chocolatiers and patisseries), and chocolate chips—when used to coat—oftentimes have a softer texture that's best if kept chilled in the refrigerator. And, it's never shiny. There are benefits to using both, and I'll let you decide what type of chocolate you choose when making chocolates and other confections. But, quality counts, so regardless of whether or not you decide to temper, be sure to seek out the best-tasting, highest-quality chocolate you can afford when chocolate making (we'll talk about tempering below).

For couverture, most chocolate over 55 percent is dairy-free, making it suitable for vegans. I like Guittard and Barry-Callebaut brands. Coppeneur Germany is a great brand for soy-free.

> Technically, there is a variety of melting or dipping chocolate available, too—sometimes sold as "Candy Melts." These are often made with weird additives and dairy, so it's best to avoid them anyway, but they are also not made with cocoa butter and therefore are not true chocolate.

TEMPERING CHOCOLATE 101

While it is simple to coat candies and other confections in melted chocolate chips, resulting in an even, soft layer of chocolate, tempering is the process that gives hardened chocolate the typical snap and shine of professional chocolates. Tempering chocolate may seem daunting, especially if you've never even heard of it, but I assure you, just like anything, with a little practice, you'll soon have perfect results. You must gather a few required ingredients and tools before attempting to temper chocolate:

1.   High-quality couverture chocolate

2.   A double boiler/bain marie or stainless steel bowl and saucepan to act as a double boiler

3.   A chocolate thermometer. Be sure to seek out a thermometer made for chocolate, or one that reaches a temperature of at least 80°F accurately and measures in small increments.

4. Patience and persistence

5. Chocolate molds (and chocolate gloves)

When you first begin tempering, you may feel nervous; rest assured, you can always let the chocolate cool and then start all over again if you've messed up. Plus, once you finally nail tempering, you will have a remarkable sense of satisfaction. The gorgeous sheen and tight snap from tempered chocolate is well worth the additional effort, which is mostly wait time.

To temper, follow these instructions, making sure never to allow any water near or around the chocolate. If water hits the chocolate, it will be ruined—even the teensiest amount—and you won't be able to ever temper it. I also recommend using a stainless steel bowl to temper rather than stoneware or glass, as the latter tends to retain heat longer, which can be problematic for tempering.

Also, keep in mind that different couverture brands and percentages of cocoa can and will have different tempering temperatures. The directions below outline a general guideline for dark chocolate, about 61 to 66 percent cocoa content.

1.   Over medium-low heat, warm about 1 to 2 inches of water in a double boiler. Place the required amount of couverture (chopped or in coins, don't grate it) into the bowl of the double boiler while the water is still cool, making sure not to get any water whatsoever on the couverture. Melt the chocolate completely, stirring occasionally and   heat   to   115–120°F.

2.   Remove from heat and let cool to about 82°F, stirring occasionally. Once at that temperature, drop about 1 teaspoon of already tempered solid chocolate (about 3 coins from the bag of chocolate you are using) into the melted couverture. Stir a lot. This is called "seeding."

3.   Place the double boiler bowl back onto medium-low and heat while stirring, until the temperature of the chocolate is increased to 88– 91°F; once in this range, remove from heat. Do not let it get above 91°F or it won't temper. Keep a close eye on the chocolate during this step as it reheats quickly.

4.   Voilà! You have tempered chocolate. If there is any remaining "seed" chocolate, remove it before dipping, coating, or molding. Once your chocolate is tempered it should set quickly (about 20 minutes) at room temperature and will appear shiny and "snappy" when bitten into. Use in molds or to coat candies, such as the Buttery Fingers or to coat the Salted Espresso Truffles. Don't place the chocolate in the refrigerator, or it will cause "bloom," which is white streaks in chocolate that form from cocoa butter separating.

CLASSIC CANDIES

LOLLIPOPS OR HARD CANDY

YIELD: 20 CANDIES

Have you ever thought to make your own lollipops? If not, now's the time! They are easy as can be and you can completely control the flavor. One trip to a craft or candy supply store and you'll have what it takes to make enough lollies to last a year! Seek out white plastic molds as they are made specifically for molding hard candies and releasing without breakage.

1 cup sugar

½ cup water

⅛ teaspoon cream of tartar

1 to 2 drops food coloring (optional)

½ teaspoon flavored oil or extract, such as lemon or cherry

- Place the plastic (white) hard candy molds onto a flat surface and place in the lollipop sticks, if you're using them. Have the molds nearby for when your sugar is ready to go.

- Over medium heat, in a 2- or 3-quart saucepan, combine the sugar, water, and cream of tartar and heat until boiling, stirring often as it cooks. Be sure to brush down the sides of the pan with a wet pastry brush once the sugar crystals mostly are dissolved. Once the mixture is boiling, stop stirring.

- Clip on a candy thermometer. Let mixture cook until the candy thermometer reaches 300°F (or Hard Crack Stage using the Cold Water Method) or until it turns from clear to a very light caramel hue.

- Working quickly, immediately stir the food coloring and flavoring into the pot. Pour the mixture into candy molds. Rap the mold lightly on flat surface to remove any air bubbles from the candy, and let the candies set until totally hardened. Pop out and place onto waxed paper. Store in airtight container for up to 1 month.

Silicone molds are the best to use, in my opinion, when making hard candies. But, white plastic molds can be used, too. I find the plastic lollipop molds release easiest when candy is still very warm, but firm.

262

ENGLISH TOFFEE

YIELD: 8 SERVINGS

This crunchy toffee is coated with decadent dark chocolate and topped with toasted nuts. If you have a nut allergy, replace with toasted sunflower or hemp seeds, which will be just as delicious, or leave them off altogether. In the unlikely event you find yourself with leftover candy, this recipe makes a fabulous mix-in to ice cream when crushed and stirred in after the ice cream has churned. Or, try it instead of chocolate chips in the Classic Chocolate Chip Cookies.

1½ cups non dairy margarine
1½ cups sugar
¼ teaspoon salt
2 cups non dairy chocolate chips
1 cup nuts (such as almonds or pecans), toasted and chopped

- Prepare a cookie sheet or jelly roll pan with enough parchment paper or a silicone mat to cover.

- Combine the margarine, sugar, and salt in a 2-quart saucepan and melt gently over medium heat, stirring often.

- Continue stirring as the mixture hits a boil, and keep cooking until the candy mixture reaches 300°F on your candy thermometer (for about 30 minutes or Hard Crack Stage if you're using the Cold Water Method). Immediately pour liquid candy mixture onto the prepared surface and spread until about ¼ inch thick. Let cool for about 3 minutes, or until slightly firm, and then carefully place the chocolate chips into an even layer on top of the hot toffee. Allow the chips to rest for about 2 minutes, and then use a silicone spatula to smooth the chocolate over the top of the toffee.

- Sprinkle with nuts and allow to cool completely. Break into bite-size pieces. Store in airtight container for up to 1 month.

BUTTERY FINGERS

YIELD: 8 SERVINGS

These irresistible candies taste just like the commercial brand, with addictively crunchy peanut butter candy layers encased in creamy chocolate. Of course, these are just as nice without the chocolate on the outside … especially when crumbled up and sprinkled on ice cream.

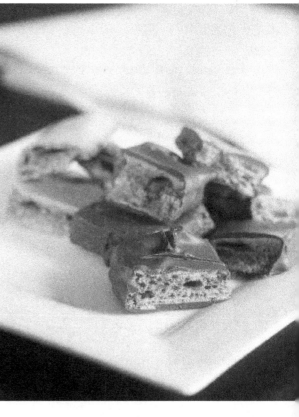

1 cup sugar
⅓ cup corn syrup
⅓ cup water, room temperature
1 cup creamy peanut butter
1 teaspoon vanilla extract
2 cups couverture, tempered (see recipe)

• Line a 9 × 13-inch baking sheet with parchment paper or have ready a silicone baking mat the same size.

• In a 2-quart saucepan combine the sugar, corn syrup, and water. Bring to a boil over medium heat, stirring often with a clean wooden spoon and washing down sides with a silicone brush. Once boiling, reduce stirring to occasionally until mixture reads 290°F on a candy thermometer (or the Soft Crack Stage if using the Cold Water Method).

• Remove from heat immediately and quickly stir in the peanut butter and vanilla extract and spread about ½ inch thick onto the baking sheet or silicone baking mat. Score lightly using a sharp knife and break into 1 × 2 inch-bars.

• Cover with tempered couverture and let the candy set until the chocolate becomes firm, for about 1 to 2 hours. Store in an airtight container for up to 1 month.

You can replace the corn syrup here with agave to make it corn-free, although the color of the candy will be darker and it may have a slightly different taste than traditional Butter-finger candy.

HONEYCOMB CANDY

YIELD: 10 SERVINGS

Whether you call it Hokey Pokey, Puff Candy, Sea Foam, Sponge Candy, or another one of its many different and amusing names, this is an especially kid-friendly candy—and a fun project for a rainy afternoon. Let the kids watch as you add in the baking soda as a super-fun surprise awaits! You'll need a large stockpot suitable for candy cooking; the candy gets BIG when you add baking soda, so make sure it's quite roomy.

¼ cup water

¼ cup agave or maple syrup

1 cup sugar

¼ cup brown sugar (dark or light)

2 teaspoons baking soda

2 cups non dairy couverture or non dairy chocolate chips, melted (see recipe)

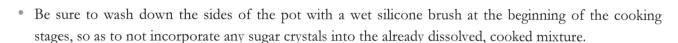

- Place a silicone mat onto a cookie sheet and set on a flat surface.

- In a stockpot thoroughly combine the water, agave, and sugars. There is no need to stir the candy while it cooks, but a nice and thorough mixing at the beginning is a good thing to do. Clip on your candy thermometer and cook over medium heat until the thermometer reaches about 285°F to 290°F, (or Soft Crack Stage using the Cold Water Method) or until the syrup darkens in color.

- Be sure to wash down the sides of the pot with a wet silicone brush at the beginning of the cooking stages, so as to not incorporate any sugar crystals into the already dissolved, cooked mixture.

- When the mixture has reached 285°F, remove from heat and quickly and carefully stir in the baking soda. It will foam up about four times its size! Stir quickly and evenly and then pour out onto the silicone mat, allowing it to freeform into a nice solid blob. Do not try to spread the mixture; just let it rest until it has cooled. Cut into bite-size squares and then cover with the chocolate. Store in airtight container for up to 1 month. If you do not wish to cover these candies, they need to be stored immediately in an airtight, dry plastic bag with all air removed (using a straw, etc.)—uncovered, the honeycomb candy will only keep a short while before changing texture.

265

CARAMELS

YIELD: 20 CANDIES

Is there anything more sinfully delicious than a chewy caramel? These sticky sweet candies will make you do flips over their authentic taste, with no need for heavy cream or butter.

1 cup sugar

1 cup canned full-fat coconut milk

½ cup light corn syrup or agave

¼ cup non dairy margarine or coconut oil

1 teaspoon vanilla extract

- Grease a baking dish or pan (or use a nonstick silicone pan). The smaller the base of the pan, the thicker your pieces of caramel will be.

- Place all ingredients, except for the margarine and vanilla extract, into a heavy 2- or 3-quart saucepan (make sure that the sides of your pan are at least 6 inches high because the caramel mixture will bubble up).

- Over medium heat, stirring constantly with a wooden spoon, dissolve the sugar completely. Next, add the margarine and stir just until boiling. Once boiling, stop stirring.

- Let the mixture continue to boil, without stirring, until it reaches 245° to 250°F on your candy thermometer (or Firm Ball Stage if you're using the Cold Water Method), which takes about 15 to 20 minutes.

- When the mixture is at the right temperature, immediately remove from heat and stir in the vanilla extract. Quickly pour into your prepared dish.

- Let cool at room temperature for a few minutes and then slip into your fridge for about an hour. Once firm, cut the caramel into squares. You can freeze the candy just for a few minutes right before cutting to make it slightly less sticky to handle.

- Wrap the candies in waxed paper and store in fridge or in cool, dry place for up to 1 month.

For an extra-special treat, try covering the firm caramels with chocolate, either couverture that has been tempered (see recipe) or melted chocolate chips. Be sure the caramels are room temperature or colder before attempting to coat with chocolate, and once dipped, place on parchment or waxed paper. Let the chocolate reharden at room temperature for about 1 to 2 hours.

HAND-PULLED TAFFY

YIELD: 40 PIECES

I encourage you to seek out a willing partner if you have one handy to help pull. Not only is it more fun, but it's a little easier on your upper body as well!

1 cup sugar

1 tablespoon cornstarch

½ cup light corn syrup

1 tablespoon non dairy margarine or coconut oil, plus more for your hands as you pull

6 tablespoons water

¼ teaspoon salt

1 teaspoon vegetable glycerin (optional—see note)

½ teaspoon orange oil, lemon oil, or other extract flavoring

- Grease a small glass baking dish and gather a candy thermometer and waxed paper. Set aside a bit of margarine or coconut oil for greasing your hands as you pull.

- Whisk together the sugar, cornstarch, corn syrup, margarine, water, salt, and glycerin, if using, in a 1-quart saucepan until no lumps remain and heat over medium heat. Stir constantly until mixture comes to a boil.

- Cook, undisturbed, just until the mixture reaches 265 to 270°F on your candy thermometer (or Soft Crack Stage if using the Cold Water Method) and then immediately remove from the heat and add the flavoring.

- Pour the liquid taffy into the greased baking dish and allow to cool for about 10 minutes, or until easy to handle. Once you know you won't burn yourself, grease your (very clean) hands and grab the taffy and form into a log. Begin to stretch and pull at the taffy, creating ropes and then folding and repulling to add air into the candy. Continue pulling for about 15 minutes, until the color has lightened significantly and feels light and airy, like taffy. Cut into bite-size pieces and then wrap individually in waxed paper. Store in airtight container for up to 1 month.

The glycerin in this recipe can be sourced from candy-making supply stores and online. It's totally optional, but it does help ensure a creamy, smooth texture to your taffy.

TURKISH DELIGHT

YIELD: 30 PIECES

Turkish Delight may be the origin of the jelly bean, with its chewy fruity center being an inspiration for the candy-covered beans. This candy is easy to prepare as long as you have all your equipment and ingredients gathered and ready to go.

MIX #1

3 cups granulated sugar

½ cup agave

½ cup water

⅛ teaspoon cream of tartar

MIX #2

1 cup cornstarch

1 cup confectioners sugar

1 teaspoon cream of tartar

2½ cups water

2 drops food coloring, any color

⅛ teaspoon lemon or orange oil, or 1 teaspoon rosewater

½ cup confectioners sugar for dusting

¼ cup cornstarch for dusting

- Grease an 8 × 8-inch baking dish. Have a sheet of cling wrap handy for covering the candy.

- In a 2- or 3-quart saucepan, combine all the ingredients for Mix #1 and bring to a boil over high heat. Once the mixture comes to a boil, reduce heat to medium and continue to cook, stirring often, until the mixture reaches 260°F (or Hard Ball Stage using the Cold Water Method). While the mixture is heating up to that temperature, move on to the next step.

- In a stockpot, whisk together the ingredients for Mix #2 (except for the food coloring and flavoring) until completely smooth and cook over medium- high heat until boiling. Once the mixture comes to a boil, cook for about 2 minutes, or until very thick. Remove from the heat.

- Once Mix #1 hits 260°F, quickly pour it into the stockpot containing Mix

#2 and stir vigorously but carefully until well combined. Reduce heat to medium low and cook for 35 more minutes, stirring often with a silicone spatula until the mixture is thick and smooth, like whipped honey.

- Add the 2 drops of food coloring and ⅛ teaspoon flavoring. Pour into prepared baking dish and cover immediately with cling wrap. Let candy firm and cool down to room temperature, for about 30 minutes.

- Whisk together cornstarch and confectioners sugar and gently coat the cooled candy square with the sugar mixture on each side. Use a sharp knife to cut the candy into bite-size squares. Store in airtight container for up to 1 month.

SUGAR NESTS

YIELD: 10 NESTS

Sugar Nests make a very fun addition to a dessert's presentation and are not as difficult as they appear. You do need to take caution when handling the hot syrup, making sure not to get any on you accidentally—as it gets *hot!* Otherwise, drizzle the sugar to your heart's content to make stunning shapes and designs. The bowls make a lovely presentation for ice cream when frozen for 10 minutes before scooping, or use as decorative additions to cakes.

2 cups sugar

½ cup water

3 tablespoons agave

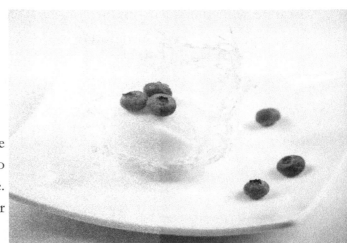

- Prepare your entire workspace by covering around the stove and on the floor with parchment, careful not to let any come too close to the burner, lest it catch fire. Keep a sheet of parchment handy for placing your finished nests.

- On one piece of parchment, flip over a large or standard-size muffin pan so you can use the bottom and outside of the cups as a mold and lightly grease the bottoms of the cups. I like almond oil, but a nonstick spray will work just fine. Secure your candy thermometer into a 2- or 3-quart saucepan. Have a large metal bowl of ice water next to you so you can be ready to dunk the pot of cooked syrup in the bowl to cool it down.

- Over medium heat, combine the sugar, water, and agave. Stirring occasionally, and brushing down the sides of the pan with a wet silicone brush to wash away any sugar crystals, cook the syrup until it reaches 310°F on your candy thermometer and turns dark amber in color (or Hard Crack Stage if using the Cold Water Method).

- Remove immediately from the heat and dunk the pot into the ice water bath. Stir briefly just until thickened and remove from the water. Using the tines of a whip-style whisk or a fork, very carefully drizzle thin strands of the hot syrup onto the greased upturned muffin tins, creating a lovely mess of strands. Set the hot sugar mixture aside on a trivet until you're ready to make the next batch of nests. Careful when working with this mixture as it is extremely hot. Use caution when handling and wear kitchen gloves if you have them.

- Let the drizzled syrup rest for about 15 seconds or until only slightly warm to the touch. Use clean dry hands to gently remove the nests from the pan and bend and form the sugar into a nest shape, or other desired form, and place onto another clean dry sheet of parchment.

- Repeat with the remaining hot sugar mixture (the mixture will remain warm in the pot). Work fast! The syrup cools quickly and you want to catch it in its perfect state of malleability and coolness to the touch.

- Use immediately for garnish or store in an airtight container for up to 1 week.

PEANUT BRITTLE

YIELD: 8 SERVINGS

Be sure to seek out raw or "Spanish" peanuts when making this recipe, as the peanuts actually cook in the hot candy mixture. If you use roasted, the peanuts will be overcooked. This candy works well with other flavors mixed in. Try 1 teaspoon cinnamon or Sriracha sauce for a fun kick.

1 teaspoon baking soda
Optional: 1 teaspoon ground cinnamon, Sriracha sauce, or other flavoring
1¼ cups raw Spanish peanuts
1 cup sugar
½ cup light corn syrup or agave
¼ cup water
1 heaping tablespoon non dairy margarine or coconut oil
1 teaspoon vanilla extract

- Grease a cookie sheet. In a small bowl mix together baking soda and cinnamon or other spice, if using. In separate container, measure out your peanuts.

- In a 2- or 3-quart saucepan, combine the sugar, corn syrup, water, and margarine. Over medium heat, stirring occasionally with a wooden spoon, bring the mixture to a boil. Once it has started boiling, add the Spanish peanuts.

- Bring back up to a boil and keep on medium heat until the candy mixture reaches 300°F on your candy thermometer (or Hard Crack Stage using the Cold Water Method).

- Remove from heat and add baking soda mixture and vanilla extract. If you are using additional flavoring, add it in now. Stir well and pour onto the greased cookie sheet. Wait a few minutes, until the candy is cool enough to handle, and pull gently to desired thickness.

- Let cool completely and then break into individual pieces. Store in airtight container for up to 1 month.

ALLERGY NOTE

For a corn-free version, use agave rather than corn syrup.

CANDY KETTLE CORN

YIELD: 5½ CUPS

Such a fun treat to serve at Halloween, or anytime! The sweet and salty combo of kettle corn is hard to resist, so be sure to double the recipe if making for a large crowd.

5½ cups popped popcorn, salted to taste (about ½ cup unpopped kernels)
2 cups sugar
1 cup light corn syrup or agave
½ cup non dairy margarine
¼ cup apple cider
1 teaspoon vanilla extract
1 teaspoon apple cider vinegar
1 cup non dairy chocolate chips
⅔ cup sliced almonds, toasted

- Make sure your popcorn is popped and set aside, ready to go in a large bowl. Have nearby a candy thermometer and a wooden spoon.

- Grease a 9 × 13-inch cookie sheet.

- In a heavy saucepan, at least 8 inches deep, combine the sugar, corn syrup, margarine, and apple cider. Over medium heat, bring the mixture to boil, stirring occasionally. Continue to cook over medium heat and stir regularly using a wooden spoon until your candy thermometer reads 300°F (or Hard Crack Stage if using the Cold Water Method). This takes a while. Patience totally pays off with these, so don't rush and pull the candy from the stove before it reaches hard crack stage. Be sure to wash down (recipe) the sides!

- Remove the candy mixture from the heat and quickly stir in the vanilla extract and vinegar. Pour HOT candy mixture over the popcorn and stir quickly until evenly coated. Let cool for about 5 to 7 minutes. Spread onto a greased cookie sheet and let cool completely.

- Using a double boiler, melt the chocolate until smooth. Drizzle melted chocolate over the candied popcorn and sprinkle with sliced almonds. Let chocolate harden and then break into bite-size pieces. Store in an airtight container in the fridge or a cool place where chocolate will not melt for up to 1 month.

PINWHEEL CANDY

YIELD: 20 PIECES

There is much speculation about the origins of this candy, ranging from German, to Irish, to Pennsylvania Dutch, to the product of ingenuity during the Great Depression when limited ingredients were all there were to work with, which may be why potatoes are a key ingredient here. Even though potatoes aren't normally thought of as dessert food, they really do work quite nicely in this recipe! I recommend using a Yukon Gold or similar variety; if you opt for russet, you may need a touch more nondairy milk to make smooth.

1 large medium-to low-starch potato, peeled, mashed, and salted lightly

¼ cup non dairy milk

1 teaspoon vanilla extract

½ teaspoon salt

2 pounds (about 6 cups) confectioners sugar (or enough to make stiff dough)

About 1 cup chocolate hazelnut butter (such as Justin's brand)

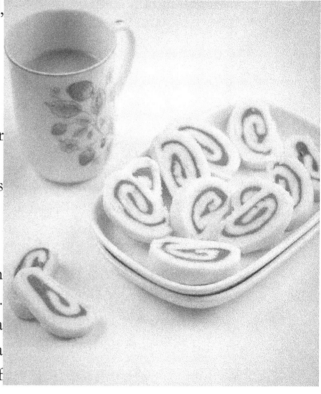

- In a large bowl, combine the mashed potatoes, non dairy milk, vanilla extract, and sea salt until smooth. Gradually incorporate the confectioner's sugar until a stiff dough forms. You may need a little more or a little less sugar depending on the moisture level of your mashed potatoes.

- Form the dough into a large patty and refrigerate for at least 2 hours. Place the chilled dough in between two sheets of plastic wrap and roll out into a rectangle about ½ inch thick. Slather generously with chocolate hazelnut butter until coated. Using the bottom piece of the plastic wrap, gently guide the dough into a roll longways as you would a jelly roll. Cover with plastic wrap and chill for an additional hour. Once chilled, cut into ½-inch-wide sections and wrap in waxed paper, twisting each side to close.

- Store in fridge in airtight container. Keeps for up to 1 week.

AFTER DINNER MINTS

YIELD: 80 MINTS

These mints are easy to whip up but impressive enough to brag about when serving to friends. Call them artisan and watch their eyes light up.

Note that you can feel free to sub in Sweet Cashew Cream for the cream cheese, just add a little more confectioner's sugar until it reaches the correct consistency.

8 ounces nondairy cream cheese
1 tablespoon non dairy margarine
2 drops pure peppermint extract/oil
Food coloring paste (use corn-free if needed)
3½ to 4 cups confectioner's sugar, plus extra for dusting (use corn-free if needed)

- Mix the cream cheese, margarine, peppermint oil, and food coloring with a whisk until smooth. Gradually add in the confectioner's sugar, about ½ cup at a time, until a stiff dough forms—much like Play-Doh.

- Pat into a disk and roll out in between two sheets of parchment paper. Cut with a very small cookie cutter (or use a knife/pizza cutter to cut into squares) into desired shapes and then place on cookie tray that will fit in your fridge. Chill for 1 hour, then transfer to a resealable plastic container to store for up to 1 month in refrigerator. These also freeze well and can be thawed in your refrigerator until eating.

MARZIPAN

YIELD: 10 SERVINGS

Sold in tiny tubes at specialty stores or in the baking aisle of your neighborhood grocery, marzipan is easy to make at home, saving you both money and the effort of finding one that is dairy-, egg- and gluten-free, which can be difficult. Bonus: almonds, the main ingredient here, are tiny powerhouses rich in calcium, iron, potassium, magnesium, copper, and zinc!

1 tablespoon flaxseed meal
2 tablespoons water
3 cups blanched almond meal
1 cup confectioners sugar, plus extra for rolling
Dash salt

- In a small bowl, combine the flaxseed meal with the water and allow to rest until thickened, for about 5 minutes.

- In a food processor, blend the 3 cups almond meal until clumpy and the texture becomes somewhat like a paste, scraping down the sides and bottom of the bowl often. It should take 7 to 10 minutes' blending time to become clumpy.

- Add the confectioner's sugar and salt and pulse until once again crumbly, for about 30 seconds to 1 minute. Drizzle in about half of the prepared flaxseed meal while the food processor is blending and continue to add a little more until the mixture clumps together into a dough. Remove from food processor and form into a cylinder. Roll out gently onto a confectioner's sugar–covered surface and then wrap tightly to store. Use immediately or keep refrigerated for up to 2 weeks.

SIMPLE WHITE CHOCOLATE

YIELD: 8 OUNCES

This confection is best used for baking or candy making, rather than straight snacking, but it's perfect for the recipes in this book that call for white chocolate. Seek out the highest-quality food-grade cacao butter you can find for top-quality flavor.

8 ounces food-grade cacao butter, chopped into ½-inch pieces
¼ cup soy milk powder
3 tablespoons agave
⅓ cup confectioners sugar
⅛ teaspoon salt
1 teaspoon vanilla extract

• In a double boiler, over medium-low heat, melt the cacao butter until completely liquefied. Whisk in the soymilk powder until completely dissolved. Stir in the agave, confectioner's sugar, salt, and vanilla extract and whisk again until very well blended with no lumps remaining. Pour straight into a plastic or silicone chocolate mold and refrigerate for 20 minutes until solid. Pop out of mold and use as desired. Store in airtight container for up to 1 month.

CHOCOLATE ALMOND NUGGETS

As a child, one of my favorite candy combinations was simply chocolate with almonds. These bite-size morsels are a tribute to these two "made for each other" flavors.

½ cup sliced almonds
1 cup non dairy chocolate
¼ cup almond meal

- Preheat oven to 375°F and spread the almonds onto a baking tray. Bake for 7 minutes, or until fragrant. Watch carefully so that they do not burn.

- Melt chocolate over a double boiler until totally smooth. Stir in the almond meal and toasted almonds. Drop by small spoonfuls onto waxed paper or a silicone mat. Let harden completely. Store in airtight container for up to 3 weeks.

EASY HOLIDAY BARK

YIELD: 8 SERVINGS

A surefire way to impress without any additional holiday stress! Add in your favorite candies from the holiday, or stick to the traditional version as I have below. Either way, you'll end up with a treat good enough to gift.

2 cups non dairy dark chocolate, coins or chips
2 cups non dairy white chocolate, chunks or chips
1 cup crushed candy canes (check ingredients for gluten or animal products)

- Have an 8 × 8-inch silicone pan ready to go. You can also use a baking sheet lined with waxed paper or aluminum foil, but silicone is best.

- Over a double boiler, melt or temper (instructions) the dark chocolate and spread evenly into the silicone baking pan. Place the chocolate in the refrigerator to firm up.

- In the meantime, prepare the white chocolate by melting over a double boiler. Depending on what type of chocolate you are using, it could be totally liquid, or very thick. Once melted, spread or pour the white chocolate on top of the solidified dark chocolate. Sprinkle with crushed candy canes. Let harden and then score into pieces. Store in airtight container for up to 1 month.

CHOCOLATE PEPPERMINT PATTIES

YIELD: 30 CANDIES

This candy takes the classic peppermint patty one step further and infuses it with an extra-intense chocolate flavor. If you cannot locate the dark cocoa powder, regular cocoa powder will work well. You can use an equal amount of Sweet Cashew Cream in place of the vegan cream cheese for a soy-free version.

2 cups confectioners sugar
¼ cup dark cocoa powder
¼ cup + 2 tablespoons non dairy cream cheese
½ teaspoon sea salt
1 teaspoon peppermint extract
2 cups non dairy semi-sweet chocolate

- In a large mixing bowl (an electric mixer works best), combine the confectioner's sugar, cocoa powder, cream cheese, salt, and peppermint extract until very smooth. Divide into two equal disks and wrap in waxed paper. Chill in the refrigerator for at least 1 hour, or for 10 to 15 minutes in the freezer.

- Place one disk of chocolate dough between two sheets of parchment and roll until about ¼ inch thick. Use a 1½-inch round cookie cutter to cut out circles. Place circles of dough back into the fridge and let chill while you melt the chocolate.

- Over a double boiler on medium-low heat, melt the chocolate until shiny and smooth, or temper according to directions on tempering. Coat the disks of chilled dough by painting on the chocolate with a pastry brush. Gently place onto a waxed paper–lined wire rack to cool. Let set until chocolate is firm. Store in refrigerator in airtight container for up to 1 month.

DOUBLE CHOCOLATE CARAMEL BARS

YIELD: ABOUT 4 CANDY BARS

These candy bars are filled with an irresistible chocolate-caramel filling that just begs you to take one more bite. These full-size candy bars can be made into small chocolate caramels by using a smaller mold. Looking for a lighter flavor? Try these with white chocolate chips in the filling instead of the three additional tablespoons of dark chocolate.

1 cup plus 3 tablespoons non dairy couverture coins or chips
2 tablespoons non dairy margarine or coconut oil
2½ cups vegan marshmallows, such as Dandies or Sweet and Sara

- Using the tempering instructions in this book, temper the 1 cup of the chocolate. Coat the inside of four standard-size candy bar molds with three-quarters of the chocolate. Let the chocolate set completely for about 1 hour.

- In a small saucepan over medium-low heat, melt the margarine along with the 3 tablespoons chocolate coins. Add in the marshmallows and stir constantly until completely melted, for about 1 to 2 minutes.

- Let cool for about 5 minutes and then fill the chocolate molds with filling. Cover with the rest of the tempered chocolate and use a straight edge to flatten completely. Let candy bars set completely, for about 2 hours, or until they easily release from the molds. Store in cool, dry place, wrapped or unwrapped in airtight container for up to 1 week.

CREAM EGGS

These are so easy to make, you just need a good chocolate mold (clear plastic) and an afternoon with nothing going on. The food coloring isn't needed in this recipe but helps create the authentic "yolk" we've grown so accustomed to in a cream egg.

1 egg-shaped plastic chocolate mold that fits twenty chocolate egg halves

2¼ cups couverture chocolate, divided

¼ cup light corn syrup

2 tablespoons non dairy margarine, softened

1 cup confectioners sugar

1 teaspoon vanilla extract

1 to 2 drops yellow food coloring

- Over a double boiler, temper 2 cups of the chocolate according to the directions on tempering. Coat the insides of twenty plastic chocolate molds shaped like egg halves. You can also use a typical truffle-style mold and coat each cavity evenly with chocolate. Let chocolate harden completely and then make the filling.

- To make the filling, in a small bowl whisk together the corn syrup, margarine, confectioner's sugar, and vanilla extract until very smooth. Transfer one-quarter of the filling into a separate bowl and add in the yellow food coloring.

- Pop out the egg shapes from the mold.

- Fill ten of the chocolate egg cavities two-thirds of the way full with the white filling and then drop a central spot of yellow fondant into the center of the white to fill almost full, leaving a little room at the top so the fondant doesn't over-flow. Temper ¼ cup of the remaining chocolate and pipe the chocolate onto just the edges of one of the eggs; use to glue each half of the eggs together, one filled and one hollow. Let chocolate harden completely. Store in cool dry place for up to 3 weeks.

TRUFFLES AND FUDGE

SALTED ESPRESSO TRUFFLES

YIELD: 36 TRUFFLES

The first chocolate truffle is speculated to have originated in France, but today, there are countless varieties from countless countries, making it one of the most popular chocolates in the world. The secret to a perfect truffle is the ratio: 2 parts chocolate to 1 part cream.

1 cup couverture chocolate or non dairy chocolate chips
½ cup canned full-fat coconut milk
⅛ teaspoon sea salt
1 teaspoon vanilla extract
½ teaspoon espresso powder
½ cup cocoa powder or almond meal, for dusting

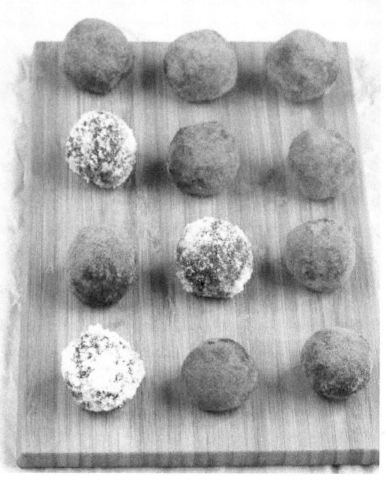

- Over a double boiler, melt the couverture until completely smooth. Remove bowl from heat and place on a heat-safe surface.

- In a small saucepan, warm the coconut milk, salt, vanilla extract, and espresso powder just until it begins to simmer and is obviously hot to the touch, but do not let it come to a boil.

- Using a whisk, gently stir the warmed coconut milk mixture into the center of the melted couverture and blend gently and carefully in a circular fashion until completely mixed. Transfer mixture to a plastic bowl and cover with plastic wrap.

- Chill in refrigerator for about 1 to 2 hours, until firm.

- Using a small scoop or rounded spoon, and chocolate-dusted hands, roll the chocolate into 1-inch balls. Immediately roll the truffles into the cocoa powder. Chill before serving and store in airtight container in the refrigerator for up to 2 weeks.

STRAWBERRY PISTACHIO TRUFFLES

YIELD: 25 TRUFFLES

What a fantastic flavor combination strawberry and pistachio make along with chocolate. Feel free to use homemade Strawberry Preserves or store-bought—both will taste equally as divine.

2 cups non dairy semi-sweet chocolate chips
¼ cup + 2 tablespoons full-fat coconut milk
1 teaspoon vanilla extract
¼ cup strawberry preserves
1 cup pistachios, chopped finely

- In a saucepan over medium-low heat, combine all of the ingredients except for the pistachios.

- Stir constantly until the chocolate is fully melted and the mixture is very well combined.

- Transfer to a bowl and chill just until it's easy to work into a ball, for about 2 hours. A quick trip to the freezer will help them out as well.

- Using a 1-inch ice cream scoop, form chocolate into balls and then roll into the chopped pistachios. Place onto a parchment-covered plate or tray and chill overnight in refrigerator or until firm. Store in airtight container in refrigerator for up to 1 month.

CHERRY CORDIALS

YIELD: 15 TO 20 CANDIES

These candies are simple to make but do require tempered couverture and chocolate molds to make them work, as untempered chocolate is too soft and no molds will cause messy cordials. For a quick refresher on how to temper chocolate, refer to tempering.

15 to 20 maraschino cherries, stems removed (see note)
¼ cup brandy
1 cup couverture, tempered
⅓ cup + 1 tablespoon confectioners sugar
3 teaspoons cherry juice (from cherry jar)
¼ teaspoon vanilla or almond extract
A chocolate mold

- Drain the liquid from the maraschino cherries, set it aside, and place the cherries on a paper towel. Transfer the cherries into a small bowl containing the brandy and allow to soak for 1 hour. Remove from brandy and place onto a dry paper towel. Let the cherries rest until they are fairly dry to the touch, for about 1 hour.

- Brush the tempered chocolate onto the insides of the chocolate mold to coat the sides evenly. Let chocolate completely harden. Place one cherry into each cavity.

- Mix together the confectioner's sugar, cherry juice, and vanilla extract and pour a small amount (just to fill) on top of the cherries. Top with tempered chocolate and let rest until chocolate has completely hardened. Store in airtight container for up to 1 week.

ALLERGY NOTE

Use vanilla extract instead of almond for a nut-free candy.

You can also omit the fondant filling and just dip the brandy soaked cherries straight into the tempered couverture. This works especially well if you leave the stems on the cherries. Just dip and place onto waxed paper to harden.

BUCKEYES

You can use chocolate chips with these or couverture. Born and raised in Ohio, I tend to think the chocolate chip method is more authentic, but, admittedly, the couverture is definitely more glamorous and adds a nice shell to the outer layer. Be sure when dipping to leave a little bit of peanut butter exposed (about ½ inch in diameter) so that the candies resemble actual buckeyes!

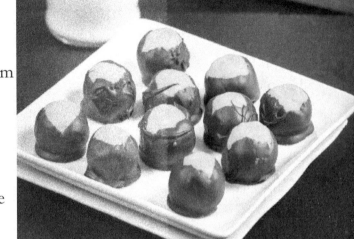

1½ cups smooth peanut butter

1 cup non dairy margarine, softened to room temperature

2 teaspoons vanilla extract

¼ teaspoon salt

5¾ to 6 cups confectioners sugar

3 cups non dairy chocolate chips or couverture

- Line a 9 × 13-inch cookie sheet with waxed paper.

- Mix together peanut butter and margarine until super smooth.

- Stir in vanilla extract and salt.

- Using electric mixer, slowly incorporate the confectioner's sugar until little crumbles form. The mixture should go from very creamy to looking like pulverized very crumbly dry cookie dough.

- Take a pinch or two of the powder/dough and, using your hands, work to form into 1-inch balls. If they appear uneven, keep working them in your hands until smooth and spherical.

- Place each onto a cookie sheet and insert a toothpick into the center. Gently pat around the toothpick to kind of "seal" it into the peanut butter ball.

- Chill in freezer for about 40 minutes, or until very firm. This prevents the toothpicks from sliding out while dipping.

- Using a double boiler, melt your chocolate until smooth or follow the directions for tempering. Remove the peanut butter balls from the freezer and carefully swirl the ball into the chocolate, taking care not to let the toothpick slide out. Place onto wax paper and repeat until all are covered.

- Let stand at room temperature until chocolate has firmed up. Remove toothpicks and seal over the tiny hole in the middle using the back of a spoon or clean fingertips. Store in airtight container for up to 1 month.

DARK AND DREAMY FUDGE

YIELD: 64 PIECES

Super rich and extra dreamy, this fudge is best enjoyed in small pieces so that you can savor the intense flavor. If you like some crunch in your fudge, simply add 1 cup of toasted walnut pieces into the fudge before spreading into a prepared pan, or sprinkle on top.

½ cup sugar

1 teaspoon vanilla extract

2 tablespoons non dairy milk

2 tablespoons non dairy margarine

10 ounces Ricemellow (vegan marshmallow) Cream

3 cups non dairy chocolate chips

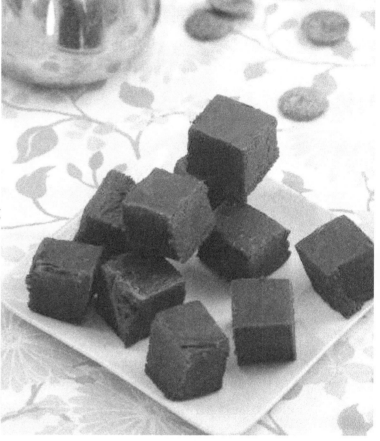

- Prepare an 8 × 8-inch pan by lightly greasing with non dairy margarine.

- In a 2-quart saucepan, combine the sugar, vanilla extract, nondairy milk, and margarine and bring to a boil over medium heat. Cook for 1 minute, stirring often. Stir in the Ricemellow Cream and heat just until warm and all of it has evenly combined with the sugar mixture, for about 4 minutes.

- Quickly stir in the chocolate chips until they have completely melted and pour the mixture into the prepared pan. Let cool completely and then chill in the refrigerator for at least 2 hours before cutting. Store in an airtight container in the refrigerator for up to 1 month.

PEANUT BUTTER FUDGE

YIELD: 20 PIECES

This is a perfect choice for when you're craving candy, but don't have a candy thermometer handy. Working quickly is an important part of making this fudge, so be sure to have all your ingredients and equipment ready before you begin.

½ cup non dairy margarine

2 cups brown sugar

½ cup non dairy milk

1 cup creamy peanut butter

1½ teaspoons vanilla extract

3 cups confectioners sugar

1½ cups non dairy chocolate chips

- Lightly grease a standard-size loaf pan or small square cake pan.

- In a 2-quart saucepan, over medium heat, warm the margarine until melted. Add the brown sugar and nondairy milk and cook over medium heat until mixture comes to a hard boil (for about 2 to 3 minutes).

- Once it comes to a hard boil, set your timer for exactly 2 minutes. Continue to cook over medium heat, stirring the entire time it is cooking, washing down sugar crystals as needed.

- After 2 minutes, remove from the heat and quickly stir in your peanut butter and vanilla extract, and promptly add the confectioner's sugar, mixing briefly just until all the sugar has been incorporated.

- Spread the thick candy into prepared pan and wait for it to set up slightly.

- Once the fudge has cooled slightly, melt chocolate chips over a double boiler and drizzle all over the fudge. Let chocolate reharden and then serve! Store in airtight container for up to 2 weeks.

FRUIT-BASED CANDIES

SUGAR PLUMS

YIELD: 24 SUGAR PLUMS

These little gems have become well known from their very important cameo in the classic Christmas tale, and, even though they may conjure up images of sugar-covered plums in your mind, they actually have never contained any plums at all. "Plum" used to be a popular way to describe any dried fruit, but sugar plums usually contained a mixture of dates, apricots, or figs to achieve their sweetness.

1 cup raw almonds
1 teaspoon lemon or orange zest
½ cup chopped dried figs
½ cup chopped dried dates
½ teaspoon cinnamon
¼ teaspoon nutmeg
Dash ground cloves
2 tablespoons agave
½ cup confectioners sugar for dusting

- Preheat oven to 400°F and spread the almonds in an even layer on a cookie sheet. Bake for 7 minutes, or until fragrant.

- Place almonds, zest, figs, dates, cinnamon, nutmeg, and cloves into a food processor and pulse until crumbly. Add in the agave, 1 tablespoon at a time, and pulse again, until the mixture comes together easily. Pinch into 1-inch balls and roll in the confectioner's sugar. Store in airtight container for up to 1 week.

ALLERGY NOTE

For a nut-free variation, try these with toasted sunflower seeds, hemp seeds, or even flaked coconut in place of the almonds.

CANDIED ORANGE PEELS

YIELD: 3 CUPS

Candied orange peels are so nice to have for decorative purposes or to add a little zing to a dessert, like in my Florentines. This recipe also works nicely with lemon or lime peels, which add a nice color variation to the mix.

4 navel oranges
1½ cups sugar
¾ cup water
Dash salt

- Remove the peels from the oranges by slicing through the peel and quartering it, without puncturing the fruit. Gently cut off the top and bottom of the orange and then carefully peel the orange peel, leaving behind the pith and fruit. Reserve pith and fruit for another use (these make fantastic juicing oranges).

- Lay one section of peel flat onto a cutting area, light-side-up. Slice the peel into thin, even strips, about ¼ inch wide.

- Place the peels into a medium saucepan and cover with 1 inch of water and salt very lightly. Boil for 20 minutes, and then drain. Briefly place onto clean kitchen towel to dry.

- Drain the saucepan and then wipe dry. Place the drained peels, sugar, water, and salt into the pot and cook over medium heat. Cook until the mixture reaches 235°F on a candy thermometer (or Soft Ball Stage if using the Cold Water Method). Spread in an even layer onto a waxed paper–covered cookie sheet or silicone mat. Let harden for 2 hours, and for up to 12 hours before transferring to airtight container. Store for up to 1 month.

SOUR FRUIT JELLIES

YIELD: 30 CANDIES

These jelly candies are a touch softer than traditional gumdrops. They actually taste more like fruit snacks made for children's lunches.

¾ cup white grape juice

⅓ cup fruit pectin

½ teaspoon baking soda

1 cup sugar

1 cup agave

1 to 2 drops food coloring, any color

¼ teaspoon citric acid

⅓ cup turbinado sugar

- Line an 8 × 8-inch pan snugly with aluminum foil and spray generously with nonstick spray or grease with margarine.

- In a small saucepan, over medium heat, warm the grape juice, pectin, and baking soda just until boiling. Once boiling, reduce heat to lowest setting, stirring occasionally.

- In a 2-quart saucepan, whisk together the sugar and agave and cook over medium heat, until it reaches 265°F on a candy thermometer (or Hard Ball Stage if using the Cold Water Method). Be sure to stir occasionally while this mixture is cooking, and, once the sugar dissolves, brush down the sides with a wet pastry brush to remove any crystals.

- After the sugar mixture has reached 265°F, stir in the grape juice mixture along with the desired shade of food coloring. You can easily separate these into various colors by pouring the mixture into separate bowls and coloring each a different color. Pour into the prepared pan (or pans if making multiple colors) and chill in refrigerator overnight. Remove from refrigerator and cut into shapes using a very small cookie cutters. Mix the citric acid and turbinado sugar in a small bowl and dip the cut candies to coat. Store in refrigerator in airtight container for up to 1 month.

Citric acid, which adds the sour flavor, can be located in most supermarkets next to canning goods. Of course, you could always leave the citric acid out and keep them sugary sweet instead.

Chapter 8

NATURE'S CANDY: REFINED SUGAR–FREE TREATS

This chapter captures the essence of sweet, without the need for any refined sweeteners. Instead, I've come up with a slew of recipes that utilize fruits and other refined sugar–free sweeteners such as maple syrup, agave, and stevia, and many of them use whole fruit, adding a few key nutrients in there for good measure. These desserts are especially good for little ones who may be craving something extra sweet, but don't need all the extra sugar. For recipes calling for Sweetened Whipped Coconut Cream, refer to the recipe and use the stevia variation.

COOKIES AND OTHER FAMILIAR FAVORITES

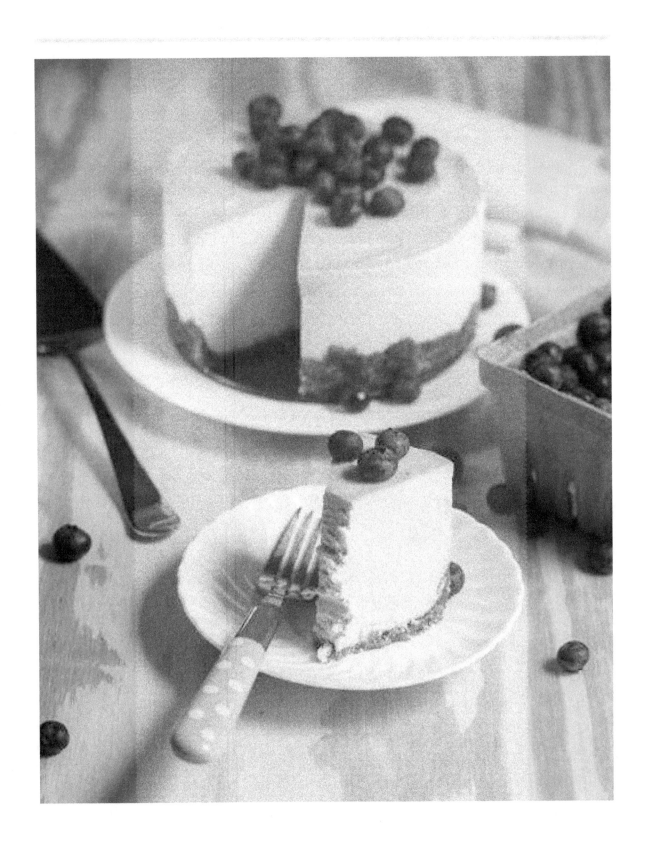

NO-BAKE CASHEW CHEESECAKE

YIELD: 10 SERVINGS

The crust on this cheesecake when made by itself can be tightly packed into 1-inch balls and devoured. These are one of my favorite treats after a strenuous hike or run. For best results, let the cheesecake rest in the fridge, covered, for 1 day before serving.

CRUST
½ cup sliced almonds
5 Medjool dates, pitted

FILLING
3½ cups raw cashews, soaked for at least 1 hour
¾ cup fresh lemon juice
⅓ cup maple syrup or agave
⅓ cup coconut sugar
1 cup organic, unrefined coconut oil, liquefied (see sidebar)
½ cup water
1 vanilla bean or 2 teaspoons vanilla extract
½ teaspoon sea salt

- Lightly grease a 6-inch springform pan using coconut oil.

- Blend the almonds and dates in a food processor until they are finely chopped and they ball together easily when squeezed. Press the mixture very compactly into the bottom of the springform pan. The bottom of a flat drinking glass works perfectly for this.

- Place all of the ingredients for the filling into a food processor and blend until smooth, for about 7 minutes, scraping down the sides as needed.

- Pour the filling on top of the crust and spread out using a silicone spatula until even. Rap on a flat surface a few times to remove any lurking air bubbles. Cover the top of the pan with foil and freeze overnight. Once frozen, transfer to the refrigerator. The cheesecake will be ready to serve after about 1 to 2 hours. Store in airtight container in freezer for up to 1 month, or refrigerate for up to 3 days.

TO MELT COCONUT OIL

Measure out 1 cup of solid coconut oil into a tall drinking glass and place in shallow bowl of hot water. As it softens, stir. Replace the water in the shallow bowl with fresh hot water and repeat until all is melted, or about 4 times to make the coconut oil reach a fully liquid state.

COCONUT CREAM TARTS

YIELD: 6 TARTS

These raw treats can be made in mini muffin pans for bite-size treats or standard-size muffin tins for larger tarts. When making raw tarts, I prefer using silicone molds as it is much easier to release the treats without breaking.

1 cup almond meal
4 Medjool dates
3 tablespoons unrefined coconut oil
½ teaspoon salt
½ teaspoon coconut extract
¾ cup Sweet Cashew Cream
⅓ cup unsweetened flaked coconut

- Place the almond meal, dates, coconut oil, and salt into a food processor and pulse until the mixture comes together easily when squeezed. Press firmly into six cups in a standard-size muffin pan, shaping into a crust with the back of a rounded spoon or using a very small bowl.

- In a medium bowl, whisk together the coconut extract and cashew cream until fluffy. Pipe into the prepared crusts and top with flaked coconut. Freeze for 2 hours and then transfer to the refrigerator. Serve cold. Store in airtight container in refrigerator for up to 1 week.

PUMPKIN MUFFINS

YIELD: 12 MUFFINS

These tender morsels are studded with raw pumpkin seeds, called pepitas, to add a delightful color and texture to the muffins.

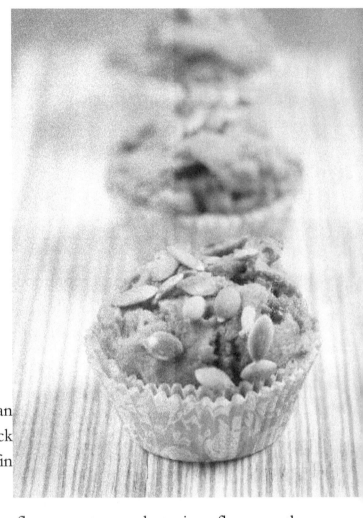

1¼ cups brown rice flour

½ cup potato starch

¼ cup tapioca flour

1 teaspoon xanthan gum

¼ teaspoon baking soda

1 teaspoon baking powder

1 teaspoon salt

1 teaspoon cinnamon

1 cup coconut palm sugar

¼ cup olive or coconut oil

1 cup pumpkin puree

⅓ cup + 2 tablespoons non dairy milk

2 tablespoons apple cider vinegar

½ cup pepitas

- Preheat oven to 400°F and line a muffin pan with twelve liners, lightly spritz with nonstick spray, or simply grease a standard-size muffin pan.

- In a large bowl, whisk together the brown rice flour, potato starch, tapioca flour, xanthan gum, baking soda, baking powder, salt, cinnamon, and coconut palm sugar. Stir in the oil, pumpkin puree, nondairy milk, and apple cider vinegar and mix until smooth. Fold in the pepitas. Divide batter evenly among the twelve cups and bake for about 20 minutes, or until a knife inserted into the center comes out clean. Store in airtight container for up to 3 days.

BANANA NUT MUFFINS

YIELD: 12 MUFFINS

These muffins are just too darn delicious with the warm flavor of banana and walnuts. Be sure to grease the muffin liners on these, or use silicone muffin cups; since these muffins contain very little oil, they may have a tendency to stick.

¾ cup brown rice flour
½ cup potato starch
¼ cup tapioca flour
1 teaspoon xanthan gum
1½ teaspoons baking powder
¼ teaspoon baking soda
¼ teaspoon salt
1 teaspoon vanilla extract
3 mashed bananas, about 1⅓ cups
⅓ cup + 1 tablespoon maple syrup
2 tablespoons olive oil
2 tablespoons vinegar
½ cup chopped walnuts

- Preheat oven to 350°F. Using margarine or coconut oil, grease twelve standard-size muffin cups, or spritz twelve liners with nonstick spray.

- In a medium bowl, whisk together the brown rice flour, potato starch, tapioca flour, xanthan gum, baking powder, baking soda, and salt. Make a well in the center and stir in the vanilla extract, bananas, maple syrup, olive oil, and vinegar. Stir the mixture until very well combined and then fold in the walnuts.

- Divide the batter evenly among the muffin cups and bake for 30 minutes, until golden brown on edges. Let cool completely before serving. Store in airtight container for up to 3 days.

These muffins take exceptionally well to a few cacao nibs added to the batter before baking.

LEMON POPPYSEED SCONES

YIELD: 12 SCONES

Scones have always intrigued me with their not quite biscuity, not quite cakey demeanor. I don't exactly want to eat them for breakfast but they always seem perfect for a midday snacking.

⅓ cup almond flour
⅓ cup corn flour
1 cup millet flour
½ cup brown rice flour
½ cup tapioca flour
1 teaspoon xanthan gum
2 teaspoons baking powder
1 teaspoon baking soda
½ teaspoon salt
½ cup nonhydrogenated vegetable shortening
½ cup maple syrup
1 tablespoon flaxseed meal
2 tablespoons water
½ cup lemon juice
2 tablespoons poppyseed
1 tablespoon lemon zest

- Preheat oven to 375°F. Mix the almond flour, corn flour, millet flour, brown rice flour, and tapioca flour together in large mixing bowl. Stir in xanthan gum, baking powder, baking soda, and salt.

- Cut in the shortening using your hands, until it forms equal-size crumbles. Add in maple syrup. In a small bowl, combine the flaxseed meal and water and let rest until thickened, for about 5 minutes.

- Using a fork, combine the prepared flaxseed meal with the rest of the ingredients until the mixture becomes evenly crumbly.

- Still using a fork, mix in the lemon juice, poppyseed, and lemon zest. Once dough becomes well mixed, turn out onto a lightly floured surface (millet flour is recommended) and gently fold over about three times. Roll about ¾ inch thick and cut into squares using a sharp knife. You can also use a biscuit cutter to make circles. Place onto ungreased cookie sheet.

- Bake for about 13 minutes or until golden brown on top. Store in airtight container for up to 1 week.

GINGERBREAD SQUARES

YIELD: 8 SERVINGS

Sweetened by banana, blackstrap molasses, and agave, this healthy gingerbread tastes just as rich and spicy as the traditional version.

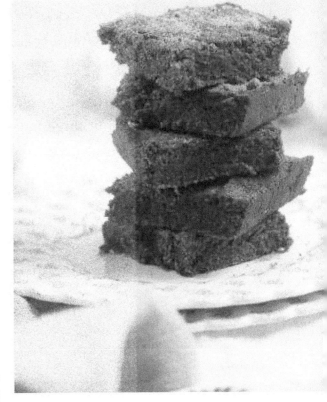

1 ripe banana, mashed

2 tablespoons blackstrap (or regular) molasses

1 teaspoon freshly grated ginger

1 teaspoon cinnamon

¼ teaspoon cloves

¼ teaspoon salt

2 tablespoons agave or maple syrup

2 tablespoons ground chia seed

1 cup almond meal

⅓ cup teff flour

• In a large bowl, stir together the banana, molasses, ginger, cinnamon, cloves, salt, and agave until smooth. Fold in the chia seed, almond meal, and teff flour. Lightly grease a 4 × 8-inch loaf pan and spread the mixture into the pan. Bake for 30 minutes. Let cool completely and then slice into squares. Store in an airtight container for up to 1 week.

SWEET CORNCAKE COOKIES

YIELD: 12 COOKIES

Corn adds a sweet touch as well as a nice color to these cookies, which can be made with maple syrup or agave. Masa harina can be found in Mexican groceries or in most grocery stores along with the Mexican ingredients.

2 tablespoons flaxseed meal
4 tablespoons water
¾ cup fine yellow cornmeal
½ cup maple syrup or agave
½ teaspoon salt
½ cup masa harina
¼ cup white rice flour
¼ cup tapioca flour
1 tablespoon olive oil

- Preheat oven to 350°F. Line a cookie sheet with parchment or a silicone mat. In a small bowl, mix the flaxseed meal with water and allow to rest until gelled, for about 5 minutes. Mix together all the ingredients in a medium bowl in the order listed, scraping sides of bowl well while mixing.

- Drop by the tablespoonful onto the prepared cookie sheet and flatten slightly with the back of a fork. Bake for 12 to 15 minutes.

- Let cool completely before serving. Store in airtight container in refrigerator for up to 1 week.

CHOCOLATE-COVERED PECAN PIE COOKIES

YIELD: 20 COOKIES

With chia seed and nuts, these delicious cookies taste sinful but are made from surprisingly wholesome ingredients. For a slightly more convenient version (and almost refined sugar–free), use non dairy chocolate chips for dipping the bottoms of the cookies instead of Raw Chocolate.

2 teaspoons ground chia seed

2 tablespoons water

1½ cups raw pecans

1 cup raw cashews

¼ cup coconut flour

½ teaspoon salt 6 dates

¾ cup Raw Chocolate, melted

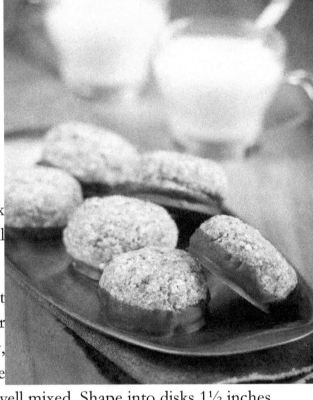

- Preheat oven to 325°F. In a small bowl, mix together the chia seed and water and let rest until gelled, for about 5 minutes.

- Place the pecans, cashews, coconut flour, and salt into a food processor and blend until crumbly, for about 1 minute. Do not overmix! Once crumbly, add the dates, two at a time, until the mixture clumps together easily. Process just until dates are well mixed. Shape into disks 1½ inches wide by ½ inch thick and place onto an ungreased cookie sheet. Bake for 15 minutes.

- Let cool and then dip bottoms of cookies into the Raw Chocolate, placing back onto a silicone mat or wax paper–covered baking sheet. Chill for about 20 minutes in refrigerator until the chocolate has set. Store in airtight container for up to 1 week.

APRICOT COOKIES

YIELD: 18 COOKIES

These golden, chewy, slightly sweet cookies are just as easy to prepare as they are to eat! Packed with vitamins A and C from the apricots and protein and iron from the walnuts and coconut, these cookies are like snack-size energy bars.

3 cups dried apricots
1 cup walnut pieces
2 cups unsweetened shredded coconut, plus about ⅓ cup for rolling
¼ cup agave

- Combine all ingredients (set aside ⅓ cup coconut) in a food processor and process until very well chopped.

- Using clean hands, roll the mixture into walnut-size balls and then into the extra coconut. Flatten into cookie rounds using the bottom of a glass or measuring cup, and then gently shape with hands to create even patties.

- Store in airtight container for up to 1 week.

CINNAMON AMARETTI

YIELD: 36 COOKIES

Amaretti are classic small Italian cookies that are crisp on the outside and a bit chewier in the center—and one of my favorite cookies of all. You won't miss the refined sugar in this version. For best texture, shape the cookies into small mounds, about 1 inch across, for perfect chewy-center-to-crispy-outside ratio.

3 tablespoons flaxseed meal
6 tablespoons water
3 cups almond meal
1½ teaspoons cinnamon
1¼ cups coconut palm sugar
¾ teaspoon salt
Sliced almonds, for garnish

- Preheat oven to 300°F. Line a large baking sheet with parchment paper.

- In a small bowl, combine the flaxseed meal with the water and let rest for 5 minutes, until gelled. Transfer to a large bowl and stir in the almond meal, cinnamon, palm sugar, and salt. Keep stirring until the mixture comes together into a stiff dough; it may not appear to be coming together, but keep stirring! This is also done effortlessly using an electric mixer.

- When the dough stiffens, pinch off 1-inch sections and form into rounds. Place onto the cookie sheet about 1 inch apart and top with a sliced almond. Bake for 30 minutes. Let cool completely. Store in airtight container for up to 1 week.

CITRUS-KISSED MACAROONS

YIELD: 18 COOKIES

Lightly touched with lemon, these macaroons have only a handful of ingredients and don't need to be baked. They make a great snack post- workout or when the midday munchies arise.

12 Medjool dates, pitted
1 tablespoon lemon juice
2 tablespoons water
4 cups unsweetened shredded coconut, divided

- Combine the Medjool dates, lemon juice, and water in a food processor and blend until very smooth, scraping down the sides as necessary. Add 1 cup shredded coconut and pulse until very well combined.

- Transfer to a large bowl and by hand incorporate the additional 3 cups coconut until evenly mixed. Form the mixture into cookies and place onto cookie sheet. Refrigerate briefly to set.

- Store in an airtight container for up to 2 weeks.

PEANUT BUTTER CHOCOLATE CHIA PUDDING

YIELD: 2 SERVINGS

This dessert is as easy as pie (or pudding) to make, and it's healthy, filling, and delicious, too. Adjust sugar levels to your taste preferences, erring on the low side of things.

3 tablespoons whole chia seed, white or black
½ cup water
2 tablespoons non dairy milk (I recommend almond or coconut)
1 tablespoon cocoa powder
3 tablespoons creamy peanut butter
1½ tablespoons coconut date syrup or maple syrup

- Place all ingredients into a small to medium bowl and stir vigorously with a fork until smooth. Transfer into desired serving dishes and chill in refrigerator until gelled, for about 30 minutes. Best if served cold with a dollop of whipped coconut cream. Keeps for up to 1 day if stored in airtight container in the refrigerator.

CHOCO-CADO PUDDING

YIELD: 4 SERVINGS

Here's another surprise ingredient from the plant world: avocado is the superstar here, making a creamy base for this insanely rich chocolate pudding.

2 ripe avocados, pitted and peeled
¼ cup Date Syrup or agave
3 tablespoons coconut sugar
¼ cup cocoa powder
½ teaspoon espresso powder
¼ teaspoon salt

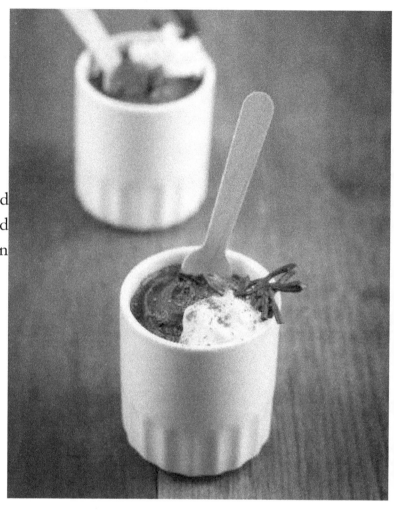

- Blend all ingredients together into a food processor until fluffy. Serve with whipped coconut cream! Store in airtight container in refrigerator for up to 3 days.

CLASSIC-STYLE SWEETS

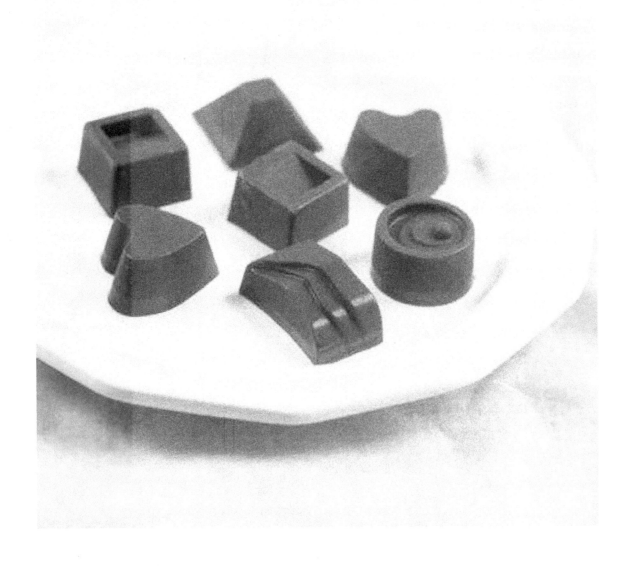

RAW CHOCOLATE

YIELD: 12 CANDIES

This chocolate can be molded using a chocolate mold or drizzled onto desserts for a chocolaty coating. Feel free to control the sweetness to your liking without affecting the final texture too much.

½ cup melted cacao butter

⅓ cup + 2 tablespoons cocoa powder

⅓ cup agave or maple syrup Pinch salt

- Whisk together all of the ingredients into a medium bowl. Pour the mixture into molds and rap on a solid flat surface to remove any air bubbles. Chill in the refrigerator until solid. To use as a coating, simply melt all ingredients back down and whisk well to combine. Store in airtight container in refrigerator for up to 1 week.

COCONUTTY CANDY

YIELD: 24 PIECES

This subtly sweet treat is nuts over coconut, in that it is made entirely out of coconut, save the vanilla extract and salt. To cut easily, let the solid candy thaw at room temperature for about 20 minutes before slicing and then returning to the refrigerator.

12 ounces (about 2½ cups) unsweetened shredded coconut
½ cup softened coconut oil, unrefined
1 teaspoon vanilla extract
½ cup coconut palm sugar
⅛ teaspoon salt

- In a blender or food processor, blend the coconut until smooth like peanut butter. This could take anywhere from 3 to 10 minutes, depending on your appliance, the dryness of the coconut, and temperature, among other factors. Just blend until smooth, and, if it never gets smooth, add a teaspoon or two of coconut oil to move things along.

- Once the shredded coconut has blended, add the remaining ingredients and blend until smooth. Pour into an 8 × 8-inch square dish, cover loosely with plastic wrap, and freeze for 30 minutes. Cut into small squares, and transfer to the refrigerator to store for up to 2 weeks.

ALMOND BON BONS

YIELD: 24 CANDIES

These are such a fun treat to snack on when a chocolate craving hits. Make a batch and store in the freezer—you can just grab one whenever you're in need of a little mood boost!

FILLING

1 cup almond meal

2 tablespoons coconut oil, softened

2 tablespoons agave, brown rice, or maple syrup

3 tablespoons melted cacao butter

⅛ teaspoon salt

COATING

1 recipe Raw Chocolate, melted

- In a medium bowl, combine all the filling ingredients and let rest for about 10 minutes. Shape into balls or place into silicone chocolate molds and then chill for about 30 minutes in the refrigerator, or for 10 minutes in the freezer, until solid.

- Once the filling is cold, dip the balls into the chocolate coating until completely covered, and then place coated truffles onto a silicone mat or parchment-covered surface to harden. Dip once more in the chocolate coating and then allow the chocolate to harden completely in the refrigerator, for about 1 hour. Store in airtight container in refrigerator for up to 1 month, or in freezer bags, tightly sealed, for up to 3 months.

RAISINETTE BONBONS

YIELD: ABOUT 20 BONBONS

These taste so much like the popular candies, it certainly won't seem like you're eating something so good for you!

1½ cups raisins
1 cup walnuts
¼ cup cocoa powder

- In a food processor, combine all the ingredients and blend until finely ground and clumped together, for about 1 minute. Roll into bite-size balls and place in refrigerator to chill for about 30 minutes prior to enjoying. Store in airtight container in refrigerator for up to 2 weeks.

NOURISHING BROWNIE BITES

YIELD: 12 SERVINGS

In terms of brownies, this version is much healthier than your typical chocolaty square, but they sure don't miss a beat taste-wise. You won't feel bad about going back for seconds with these, as they are packed full of healthy stuff like dates, which contain fiber; cashews, which are high in magnesium; and cocoa, which is high in iron.

10 Medjool dates, chilled in fridge
2 cups whole cashews, unroasted
2 tablespoons cocoa powder
½ teaspoon salt
2 teaspoons vanilla extract

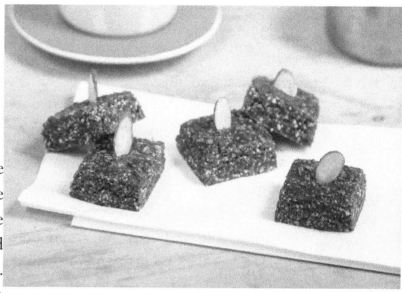

- Remove the pits from the dates and place into a food processor along with the cashews, cocoa powder, and salt. Pulse several times to combine and then blend until very crumbly, for about 2 minutes. Once the mixture is evenly crumbly, with the consistency of a coarse sugar, drizzle in the vanilla extract and continue to blend until the mixture becomes clumpy.

- Depending on the size and moisture content of your dates, you may need to add a touch more liquid, such as water or more vanilla extract, or process for a shorter amount of time to get the right consistency. In the end, the dough should easily stick together when balled. If it is too dry, add a bit more liquid (½ teaspoon or so) and if it is too wet, add in a tablespoon more cocoa powder to dry it out.

- Place the dough into the center of a parchment paper and cover with another sheet. Roll out gently to flatten into an even shape and then cut into squares. Chill in refrigerator for at least 20 minutes before serving. Store in airtight container in refrigerator for up to 2 weeks.

COOKIE DOUGH BITES

YIELD: 16 SERVINGS

A perfect pick-me-up for after dinner, or for a quick bit of fuel on the run, these little morsels taste just like raw cookie dough.

1½ cups raw cashews
9 soft Medjool dates
2 teaspoons vanilla extract
⅓ cup almond meal
Dash salt
2 tablespoons cacao nibs

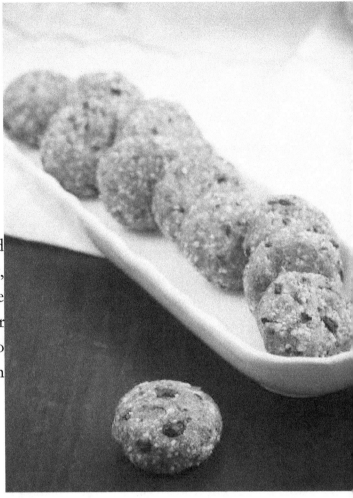

- In a food processor, pulse the cashews and dates until crumbly. Add in the vanilla extract, almond meal, salt, and cacao nibs and pulse until finely ground and dough comes together easily when pinched with fingers. Shape into small balls about 1 inch in diameter. Store in airtight container for up to 2 weeks.

PEANUTTY CHOCOLATE FUDGE BITES

YIELD: 20 CANDIES

Like the other energy bites and bars offered here, these little bits are flavor powerhouses.

½ cup cacao butter
⅓ cup + 2 tablespoons cocoa powder
⅓ cup maple syrup
3 tablespoons creamy peanut butter
Pinch salt

- In a double boiler, melt the cacao butter until liquid. Whisk in the rest of the ingredients and pour into chocolate molds or paper liners set into a muffin tin. Place in your freezer and chill for 1 hour. Pop out of molds and place onto a flat serving dish. Keep refrigerated for firmer chocolates, or store in airtight container in cool location for up to 2 weeks.

PEANUTTY CHOCOLATE FUDGE BITES

CHOCOLATE NANAIMO BARS

YIELD: 16 SERVINGS

Nanaimo bars, named after the city in British Columbia, are a popular no- bake dessert that are typically made with a LOT of butter and sugar. If you're not concerned about them being totally sugar-free, you can also use your favorite non dairy chocolate chips/buttons in place of the raw chocolate.

CRUST

1 cup whole raw almonds

10 dates

1 tablespoon cocoa powder

FILLING

2 cups cashews, soaked 2 hours

1½ teaspoons vanilla extract

⅔ cup coconut oil, melted

1 teaspoon stevia powder

3 Medjool dates or ¼ cup Date Syrup

2 tablespoons coconut cream (from the top of a chilled can of coconut milk)

TOPPING

1¼ cups Raw Chocolate, melted

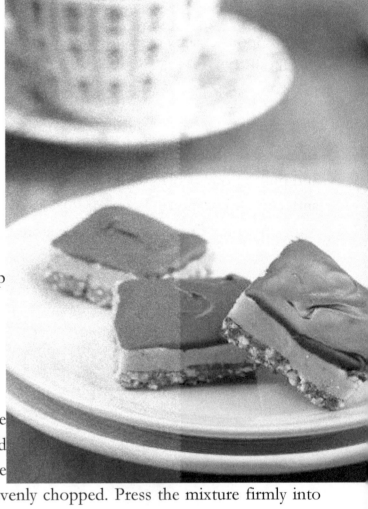

- To make the crust, in a food processor, pulse together the almonds, five of the dates, and the cocoa powder until crumbly. Add in the remaining five dates and pulse again until evenly chopped. Press the mixture firmly into an 8 × 8-inch baking pan.

- Make the filling in a food processor by combining the cashews, vanilla, coconut oil, stevia, dates, and coconut cream until very smooth, for about 5 minutes, scraping down sides as needed. Spread the filling evenly on top of the crust by using a flat silicone spatula. Freeze for 1 hour and then cut into squares.

- Top with melted chocolate and then return to freezer. Chill in freezer overnight, or for at least 6 hours. Store in refrigerator in airtight container for up to 2 weeks.

SNACK BARS AND GRANOLA

CHOCOLATE GRANOLA

YIELD: 3 CUPS

This versatile granola is perfect for all sorts of treats: Use for parfaits or to top your favorite non dairy yogurt or ice cream. Great in a bowl as breakfast cereal at home, or as a chocolaty addition to your trail mix when you're on the go.

2 cups certified gluten-free oats

⅓ cup almond meal

3 tablespoons whole chia seed

¼ teaspoon salt

⅓ cup cocoa powder

1 tablespoon coconut oil

1 teaspoon vanilla extract

⅓ cup agave or maple syrup

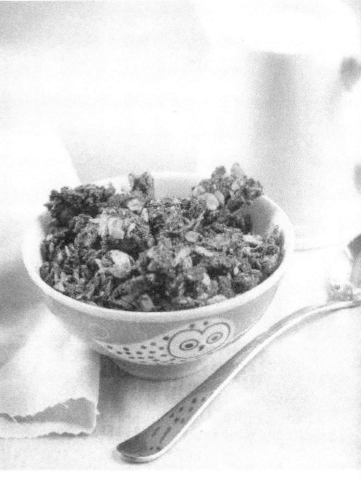

- Preheat oven to 300°F. In a medium bowl, whisk together the oats, almond meal, chia seed, salt, and cocoa powder. In a smaller bowl, whisk together the coconut oil, vanilla extract, and maple syrup until very smooth. Using clean hands, or a large fork, combine all ingredients until well mixed. Spread onto a parchment-lined jelly roll pan and bake for 40 minutes. Break into bite-size pieces and let cool completely. Store in airtight container for up to 3 weeks.

SWEET, SALTY, AND SOFT GRANOLA BARS

YIELD: 12 BARS

With its salty, sweet flavor and soft, chewy texture, this snack can satisfy multiple cravings at once! Store in an airtight container in the refrigerator for best texture.

2½ cups certified gluten-free oats

½ cup almond meal

1 teaspoon salt

2 tablespoons maple syrup

⅓ cup agave

¼ cup + 2 tablespoons softened coconut oil

¼ cup date sugar or coconut palm sugar

1 teaspoon vanilla extract

½ cup sliced almonds

1 tablespoon ground chia seed

3 tablespoons water

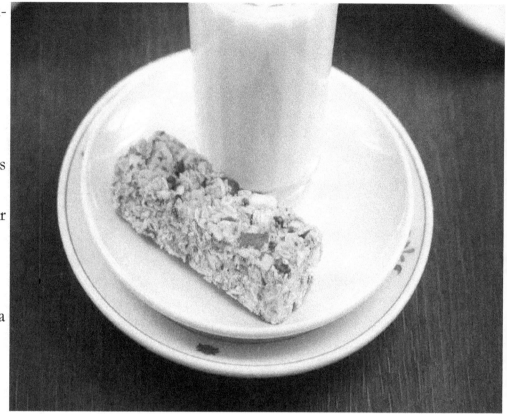

- Preheat oven to 350°F. Lightly grease an 8 × 8-inch pan.

- Spread the oats in an even layer onto a large baking sheet and lightly toast for 7 minutes. Remove oats from the oven and place them in a large mixing bowl. Using your hands, crumble in the almond meal, salt, maple syrup, agave, coconut oil, date sugar, vanilla extract, and sliced almonds.

- Mix the chia seed and water and let rest for 5 minutes, until gelled. Mix in with the rest of the ingredients and then using hands lightly greased with coconut oil, press the mixture tightly and firmly into the pan. Cover lightly with plastic wrap and refrigerate for 2 hours. Gently cut into bars and store chilled in airtight container for up to 2 weeks.

POWERHOUSE BARS

YIELD: 10 BARS

With goji berries, hemp seeds, chia seed, and oats, these protein-packed bars are full of all kinds of nourishing ingredients that will keep you going strong all day long.

1 cup pecans
½ cup raw cashews
9 dates
¼ teaspoon salt
1 tablespoon coconut oil
½ cup certified gluten-free oats
½ cup goji berries
¼ cup hemp seeds
¼ cup chia seed

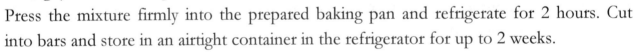

- Line an 8 × 8-inch baking pan with plastic wrap or lightly oil with coconut oil.

- Place the pecans, cashews, and five of the dates into a food processor and blend until evenly crumbly. Add the salt and the remaining dates and pulse until well combined and dates are evenly chopped. Transfer mixture into a large bowl and stir in the coconut oil to evenly coat. Fold in the oats, goji berries, hemp seeds, and chia seed. Press the mixture firmly into the prepared baking pan and refrigerate for 2 hours. Cut into bars and store in an airtight container in the refrigerator for up to 2 weeks.

CHERRY PIE BARS

YIELD: 8 SERVINGS

The taste is just like cherry pie but these little bars are actually pretty good for you! I recommend seeking out the highest-quality dried cherries (organic, unsulphured, with no added sugar) for these for the most authentic cherry-pie flavor.

2 cups raw cashews
1 cup dried cherries (not sweetened)
½ teaspoon salt
10 Medjool dates

- In a food processor, combine the cashews, cherries, and salt and blend until coarsely crumbled. Add in the dates and pulse until finely crumbled and the mixture easily comes together and stays together when squeezed.

- Shape the mixture into individual bars by shaping into a tight disk, or square, and then cutting gently with knife. Wrap individually in plastic wrap or foil. Alternatively, shape into balls for bite-size snacking. Store in airtight container in refrigerator for up to 2 weeks.

CHERRY CHOCOLATE ALMOND SNACK BARS

YIELD: 12 SERVINGS

Like a crunchy granola bar, these chocolate bars are a great pick-me-up when your energy is down. Be sure to use only kasha (toasted buckwheat) that is brown in color, rather than greenish. Kasha is usually located next to untoasted buckwheat groats, oftentimes in the bulk or natural foods sections.

1½ cups kasha (toasted buckwheat kernels), soaked for 2 hours
⅓ cup + 2 tablespoons cocoa powder
2 tablespoons chia seed
½ cup maple syrup
3 tablespoons date sugar
⅔ cup almond flour
½ teaspoon salt
½ cup dried cherries (not sweetened)
¼ teaspoon coconut or olive oil

- Preheat oven to 300°F. Line a baking tray with parchment paper.

- Drain the soaked kasha completely. In a large bowl, combine all of the ingredients except for the oil. Use the ¼ teaspoon coconut oil to grease clean hands and gently pat down the mixture into a rectangle, about ¼ to ½ inch thick. Bake for 30 minutes. Remove from oven, gently cut into squares using a spatula (but don't separate) and continue to bake for an additional 20 minutes. Let cool completely and then break into individual bars. Store in airtight container for up to 1 week.

If you can't locate toasted kasha, you can always toast your own at 300°F for 45 minutes, stirring often until browned.

FRUITY TREATS

PEANUT BUTTER BANANA ICE CREAM

YIELD: 2 CUPS

This recipe couldn't get any easier with only four ingredients, and it's good for you! Eat up.

5 very ripe bananas, peeled
½ cup smooth salted peanut butter
½ teaspoon vanilla extract
1 cup canned full-fat coconut milk

- Place all ingredients into a blender and blend until very smooth, for about 1 minute. Pour into the bowl of your ice cream maker and process according to manufacturer's instructions. Or, alternatively, freeze all ingredients in a bowl for 3 hours, and then immediately process in a food processor until smooth. Store in airtight container in freezer for up to 1 month.

FRESH FRUITSICLES

YIELD: ABOUT 5

These gorgeous pops will have you excited about eating fruit and keeping cool at the same time. I like the combo of the fruits listed below, but, along with the grapes, you could add in any chopped fruits you please. You'll need popsicle molds for these, or you can pour into silicone ice cube trays or even small paper cups.

1 cup grapes, red or green
1 kiwi, peeled and diced
⅓ cup chopped red raspberries
⅓ cup blueberries

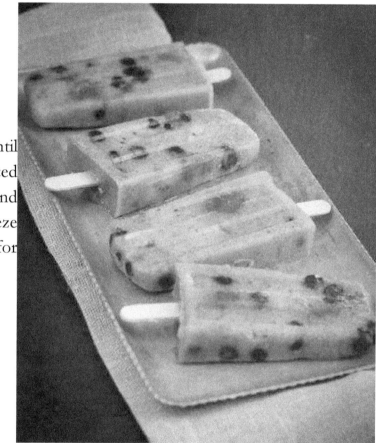

- Place the grapes into a blender and puree until smooth. Transfer to a bowl and stir in the diced fruit. Pour the mixture into popsicle molds and add wooden sticks to the center. Freeze overnight and then enjoy. Store in freezer for up to 1 month.

FRUIT SALSA AND CINNAMON CRISPS

YIELD: 6 SERVINGS

A fun twist on an old favorite, serve these "chips and salsa" at your next gathering for a sweet—and healthy—surprise.

CINNAMON CHIPS

4 white corn tortillas
1 tablespoon olive oil
1 tablespoon agave
¼ teaspoon salt
¼ teaspoon cinnamon, or to taste

FRUIT SALSA

1 cup berries (raspberry + blackberry works great)
1 cup strawberries, greens left on
½ cup seedless grapes, any variety
Juice of 1 lime
1 apple, diced with seeds removed
1 kiwi, peeled and diced

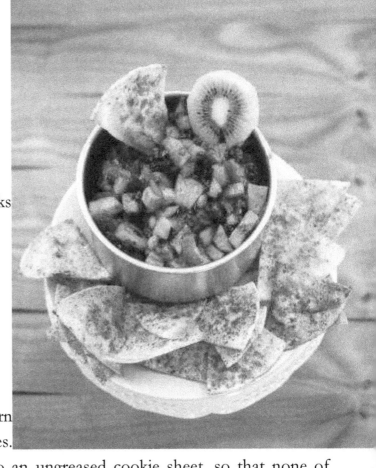

- Preheat oven to 400°F. Stack the corn tortillas and cut into six even triangles. Spread the triangles in an even layer onto an ungreased cookie sheet, so that none of them are touching.

- In a small bowl, whisk together the olive oil, agave, and salt. Brush lightly onto each side of the tortilla triangle (this will get a little sticky) and sprinkle one side of the triangles with cinnamon. Bake for 7 minutes, flip, and bake for an additional 2 minutes. Let cool while you make the salsa.

- In a food processor, combine the berries, strawberries, grapes, and lime juice and pulse until the fruit has been chopped, but not pureed, for about five or six times. Combine with the diced apples and kiwi and serve with cinnamon crisps. Store in airtight container in refrigerator for up to 1 week.

RASPBERRY CHIA JAM

YIELD: 1½ CUPS

Chia seed takes the wheel and adds an incredible thickness to this jam—no need for pectin! Use just as you would your favorite jam, and feel good about all the extra nutrients (like calcium and omega-3s) you're enjoying while doing so. If raspberry's not your favorite, practically any berry will work well using this method. Try it with blueberries, blackberries, or a mix!

1½ cups red raspberries
2 to 3 tablespoons agave, or to taste
1 tablespoon chia seed

- Place the raspberries and agave into a small saucepan and cook over medium-low heat until liquidy. Stir in chia seed and continue to cook one more minute, until thickened. Transfer to a resealable container and let cool at room temperature before transferring to the refrigerator. Store in airtight container in refrigerator for up to 2 weeks.

FRUIT AND AVOCADO SALAD

YIELD: 6 SERVINGS

Did you know that avocado is actually a fruit? That must be why it pairs so well with bananas, strawberries, and pineapple. Try it in this creamy fruit salad and see if you agree that these four were meant to be (along with blueberries and pomegranate seeds!).

SAUCE

2 tablespoons pineapple juice

2 tablespoons full-fat coconut milk

Dash cinnamon

½ teaspoon vanilla extract

FRUIT

1 large banana, sliced

4 strawberries, sliced

¼ cup diced pineapple

¼ cup blueberries

¼ cup pomegranate seeds

1 avocado, cut into bite-size pieces

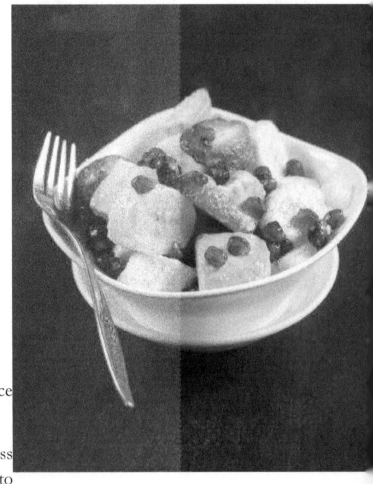

- In a small bowl, whisk together the sauce ingredients.

- Place the fruit into a medium bowl and toss with the sauce. Serve chilled. Keeps for up to 1 day if stored in airtight container.

PINEAPPLE "LAYER CAKES"

YIELD: 2 PERSONAL-SIZE CAKES

These little stacks are a fun twist on the conventional version of the dessert. Handle the pineapple rings with care, if using canned, or cut a little on the thick side if using fresh. Looking for some crunch? Try adding a thin layer of crushed walnuts or pecans on top of the cashew cream! You can locate vanilla bean paste in specialty shops such as Williams Sonoma, or simply sub in the same amount of vanilla extract.

8 pineapple rings
½ cup Sweet Cashew Cream
½ teaspoon vanilla bean paste
2 tablespoons Cherry Vanilla Compote

- Drain the pineapple rings by placing them in a single layer on a paper towel. Let rest for 10 minutes, or until the rings are relatively dry. In a small bowl, mix together the cashew cream with the vanilla bean paste.

- On the plate you wish to serve it, create an alternating stack of pineapple, cashew cream, pineapple, etc., finishing with a dollop of the Cherry Vanilla Compote.

APPLE NACHOS

YIELD: 4 SERVINGS

These are perfect for creating other variations!

3 crispy and slightly tart apples, such as Honeycrisp or Granny Smith
1 teaspoon lemon juice
3 tablespoons creamy peanut butter
¼ cup Date Syrup
¼ cup sliced almonds
¼ cup pecans, roughly chopped
¼ cup flaked or shredded unsweetened coconut
¼ cup cacao nibs

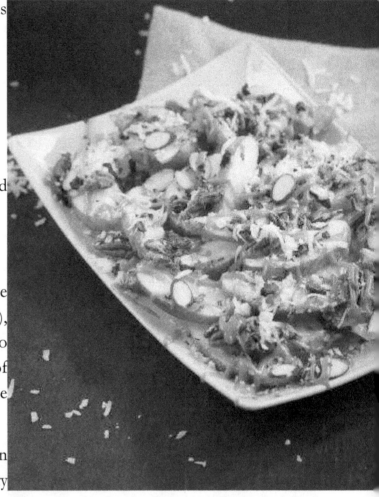

- Remove the core from each apple and slice them very thin (about ⅛-inch thickness), using a sharp knife. Arrange on a plate so that each apple has a good amount of surface exposed. Lightly spritz with the lemon juice.

- Melt the peanut butter in a small saucepan along with the date syrup until it is very runny and drizzle it onto the apple slices. Top the apples and peanut butter with the almonds and pecans, and then drizzle with the melted date syrup. Finally, top with unsweetened flaked coconut and cacao nibs. Enjoy these with your hands, just like real nachos. Serve immediately.

ALLERGY NOTE

To make nut-free, sub in toasted sunflower seeds for the almonds.

STRAWBERRY BANANA FRUIT LEATHER

YIELD: 6 SERVINGS

My kids go bananas for these wholesome snacks. I recommend using a dehydrator for best results, but you can also bake them in the oven at 200°F, spread out on a silicone mat, for several hours until dried.

2 medium very ripe (a few brown spots is desired) bananas
2 heaping cups fresh small strawberries, greens on

- Blend the fruit until smooth in a high-speed blender or food processor, scraping down sides as needed. The consistency should resemble a fruit smoothie. Spread out into a fruit leather mat fitted for your dehydrator. Spread thinly and evenly and then rap the tray on a flat surface a few times to remove any air bubbles.

- Set your dehydrator to 135°F and let it roll until the fruit is no longer tacky, for about 4 to 5 hours. If using a conventional oven, simply spread thinly onto a silicone mat and set oven to lowest temperature with the door slightly ajar. Bake for 3 to 4 hours, until no longer tacky.

- Gently peel up from the tray and place onto a cutting board. Using a pizza cutter, slice into large sections and then immediately roll up onto waxed paper, so that the fruit is completely covered. Enjoy immediately or store for up to 1 month in an airtight container.

SHAKES AND OTHER DRINKS

CARROT CAKE SMOOTHIE

YIELD: 2 SERVINGS

Indulge at breakfast time with this delish drink! It boasts the addition of blackstrap molasses, which is chock full of good stuff like copper, iron, calcium, and potassium.

1 large carrot, stems and top removed
1 large banana, peeled and frozen
3 dates
½ cup unsweetened almond milk
¾ cup cold water
½ teaspoon cinnamon
Dash nutmeg
Dash cloves
1 teaspoon blackstrap molasses

Place the first four ingredients in a blender and process until the banana is mostly blended. Add the water, spices, and molasses and blend until creamy. Thin to taste with additional cold water, if desired. Serve immediately.

PIÑA COLADA

YIELD: 2 SERVINGS

This tastes so authentic you may expect to feel a bit tipsy while sipping; but, rest assured, this libation is quite good for you. It may even ward off colds with all that pineapple, which is very high in vitamin C!

1 large peeled frozen banana
⅛ cup coconut cream (from can of coconut milk)
4 pineapple rings (or about ½ cup canned pineapple)
¾ cup pineapple juice
1 teaspoon rum extract

- Blend all ingredients until very smooth in a high-speed blender. Serve immediately.

HAPPY HEALTHY HOT COCOA

YIELD: 2 SERVINGS

This hot cocoa will leave you feeling happy and healthy after sipping as it's sweetened with date sugar and stevia, rather than the usual refined sugar mixture. I like this best made with unsweetened almond milk.

3 tablespoons cocoa powder
¼ cup date sugar
¼ teaspoon pure liquid stevia
1 teaspoon vanilla or almond extract
1 cup unsweetened non dairy milk, plus more to thin

- In a blender, combine the cocoa powder, date sugar, stevia, vanilla extract, and ½ cup almond milk. Blend on high speed until very smooth, adding the additional ½ cup almond milk as it becomes more blended. You should have a very thick, creamy, chocolate syrup.

- Thin with a little more non dairy milk until desired consistency and heat over medium heat, until warm, stirring constantly. For an extra-special treat, top with Sweetened Whipped Coconut Cream, stevia version. Serve immediately.

APPLE PIE MILKSHAKE

YIELD: 1 SERVING

Easier than apple pie, and good for you, too! This "milk shake" makes a perfectly indulgent breakfast or a late afternoon snack.

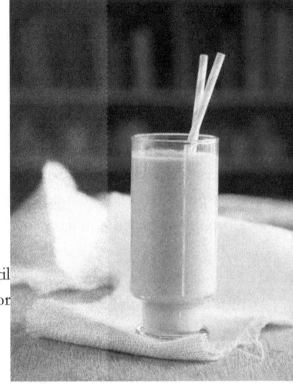

1½ bananas, chopped and frozen

⅔ cup apple cider (no sugar added)

⅓ cup pecans

½ teaspoon cinnamon

Dash nutmeg

- Combine all ingredients into a blender and mix until very smooth. Thin with a little extra apple cider or nondairy milk if desired.

- Serve immediately.

BLUEBERRY BLIZZARD MILKSHAKE
YIELD: 1 SERVING

Blueberries are full of antioxidants and lend a beautiful blue hue to this milk shake. And that's not the only healthy ingredient: it's sweetened with bananas.

½ cup fresh or frozen blueberries
1½ peeled and frozen bananas
1 teaspoon vanilla extract
1 cup non dairy milk (almond is best)

• Place all the ingredients into a blender and blend until completely smooth. Serve immediately with a thick straw.

METRIC CONVERSIONS

The recipes in this book have not been tested with metric measurements, so some variations might occur.

Remember that the weight of dry ingredients varies according to the volume or density factor: 1 cup of flour weighs far less than 1 cup of sugar, and 1 tablespoon doesn't necessarily hold 3 teaspoons.

General Formula for Metric Conversion

Ounces to grams	multiply ounces by 28.35
Grams to ounces	multiply ounces by 0.035
Pounds to grams	multiply pounds by 453.5
Pounds to kilograms	multiply pounds by 0.45
Cups to liters	multiply cups by 0.24
Fahrenheit to Celsius Fahrenheit	subtract 32 from Fahrenheit temperature, multiply by 5, divide by 9 Celsius to multiply Celsius temperature by 9, divide by 5, add 32

Volume (Liquid) Measurements

1 teaspoon = ⅙ fluid ounce = 5 milliliters

1 tablespoon = ½ fluid ounce = 15 milliliters 2 tablespoons = 1 fluid ounce = 30 milliliters

¼ cup = 2 fluid ounces = 60 milliliters

⅓ cup = 2⅔ fluid ounces = 79 milliliters

½ cup = 4 fluid ounces = 118 milliliters

1 cup or ½ pint = 8 fluid ounces = 250 milliliters

2 cups or 1 pint = 16 fluid ounces = 500 milliliters

4 cups or 1 quart = 32 fluid ounces = 1,000 milliliters

1 gallon = 4 liters

Oven Temperature Equivalents, Fahrenheit (F) and Celsius (C)

100°F = 38°C

200°F = 95°C

250°F = 120°C

300°F = 150°C

350°F = 180°C

400°F = 205°C

450°F = 230°C

Volume (Dry) Measurements

¼ teaspoon = 1 milliliter

½ teaspoon = 2 milliliters

¾ teaspoon = 4 milliliters 1 teaspoon = 5 milliliters
1 tablespoon = 15 milliliters

¼ cup = 59 milliliters

⅓ cup = 79 milliliters

½ cup = 118 milliliters

⅔ cup = 158 milliliters

¾ cup = 177 milliliters 1 cup = 225 milliliters
4 cups or 1 quart = 1 liter

½ gallon = 2 liters 1 gallon = 4 liters

Linear Measurements

½ in = 1½ cm   20 inches = 50 cm

1 inch = 2½ cm

6 inches = 15 cm

8 inches = 20 cm

10 inches = 25 cm

12 inches = 30 cm

CPSIA information can be obtained
at www.ICGtesting.com
Printed in the USA
BVHW012339260221
601199BV00008B/434